1940s HAIRSTYLES

DANIELA TURUDICH

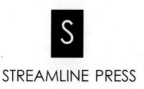

STREAMLINE PRESS

Published by Streamline Press
1535 E. 3rd Street
Long Beach, California 90802
 www.streamlinepress.com
customerservice@streamlinepress.com

First Edition
ISBN 1-930064-01-2

Edited by Glenn Soberman

Other fine books from Streamline Press are available from your local bookstore or direct from publisher.

EVERY EFFORT HAS BEEN MADE to trace and acknowledge all copyright holders. Streamline Press and the author would like to apologize if any credit omissions have been inadvertently made. If brought to our attention, we will gladly make changes to any subsequent editions.

Distributed to the book trade by IPG, Chicago.

Printed in CANADA

Thank you to all the people who gave and are still giving huge and unending amounts of constructive criticism, to my family whose never ending phone calls showed much support and love, to my answering machine who saved me from those millions of loving phone calls, to james who kept me company throughout the day...

... and finally, thank you to the my sarcastic, loving, and patient editor and soon to be husband, without whom, life would be a very boring thing.

CONTENTS

INTRODUCTION

Hair has always been a woman's most versatile accessory. Throughout history woman have always taken great lengths to style their hair to make them look more attractive.

BUT… it's the 1940s woman who, without a doubt, first mastered the art of keeping her hair in place while breaking a sweat.

The 1940s woman during the beginning of the decade worked to support the war effort. She joined the armed forces, helped sell war bonds, or wielded heavy machinery – and she looked good while doing it. Looking good and not letting her appearance falter was considered as important to the war effort and maintaining a fighting man's morale as building airplanes and organizing scrap drives. The war and safety came first, but beauty was always a close second.

It was during this time that the 1940s woman had to become creative with her hairstyling. Busy and short on time, she needed a versatile hairdo that could be styled without much fuss, while still appearing feminine. Hair was cut short, permed, and styled in waves or curls. Short hair offered easy manageability and allowed her freedom from having her hair set and styled at the salon each week. Short crops looked professional, were safely away from spinning machinery, looked good under a cap, and allowed her an evening look with just a flip of the comb.

After the war and with some extra time on her hands, the 1940s woman was again able to spend time fussing about with her appearance. Hair was left to grow longer. Styles became more loose, feminine and flattering.

She lasted this way until the end of the decade when Christian Dior brought in the New Look. Hair again was cut short to fit the new dress lines and took the 1940s women into the next decade.

This book was written for all women that find a little bit of beauty and sophistication in the hairstyles of the 1940s. It's written by a regular girl for a regular girl. All of the tips, instructions, and remedies (except for the modern method instructions) have been compiled from period sources so they are authentic in nature. The modern method instructions have been developed by consulting with professional hairdressers and as always … age-old trial and error.

Daniela Turudich

HOW TO USE THIS BOOK

This is a regular girl's guide to creating 1940s hairstyles. It uses basic techniques and practices that someone can replicate at home with a little bit of practice. I should warn you that the first time you try some of the techniques and styles, it will not come out looking as planned. It's going to take a little bit of practice, patience, and elbow grease to get a good looking style. Once you've gotten the basic techniques down, you'll be able to whip up any period do in a matter of minutes.

The most important thing to remember while reading this book is that it's meant to be an idea guide. If you don't like a style or it doesn't work for you, by all means modify it. The goal is to find a period hairstyle that works for you and brings out your best features.

The book begins with period 1940s haircutting guidelines. A period haircut is not needed to do a 1940s hairstyle, but will really make a difference if you would like to maintain an authentic 1940s look. On the opposite end, if you decide to get a period haircut, in no way does that mean that your hair will only go into 1940s styles. All of the haircutting guides encompass layers that can be quickly modified to assume a more modern styling. Unless you are an experienced hairstylist, I suggest you have a professional do the cutting.

Next up are the typical period hairstyle elements. This is the most important section of the book. This is where you figure out how to make waves, pin curls, rolls, etc. using both period and modern day methods. Really take your time in learning the various techniques. A little bit of extra time and practice will really show up in your finished hair do.

Lastly I've tried to add a variety of complete styles to choose from so that you can find what works for you. Many of the hairstyles pictured in this book have accompanying illustrations of pin curl sets, but some of them don't. If you have any questions regarding the complete hairstyles and how to do them, instructions for each element can be found in the basic elements section of the book. Remember any style can be modified or mixed and matched to come up with a style that looks good on you.

CHAPTER ONE

BASIC HAIRCUTS

1940s hairstyles require haircuts which have layers upon layers to work with. The less layers, the flatter the style, the less period the look (unless you are going for the sleek long mane like Veronica Lake). You do not have to have a period haircut in order to create a period look; however period cuts lend themselves to the styles of the period more. Nevertheless, all you really need is good, layered cut.

There are six basic haircuts from the 1940s that lend themselves to the fabulous hairstyles of that era. Instructional guides for these haircuts are provided within this chapter. Take them to your stylist or try them at home.

Important notes regarding various haircuts:
*   The lengths of hair in the shingle and shingle plus haircuts are exactly the same behind both ears.

*   The length of hair behind both ears for the baby, middy, middy plus, and long haircut is four inches.

*   For haircuts shingle plus, middy, middy plus, long, the back of the hair makes a "u" shape as it curves toward the ears. This shape was very flattering for most women and was much in demand.

Be sure to check out the combination haircuts on page 8 for other variations and options.

THE SHINGLE
VERY SHORT

The shingle haircut is about 2 inches long with a soft-feathered neckline. A modern version of this cut would be the pixie or short boyish cuts. Since the hair is very short in this cut, most styles are going to be very close to the head. Pin curl sets and wisps would look very cute here and add some style.

IMPORTANT NOTE

Period styling requires that the top hair be left longer (4 – 6 inches) so that it can be curled, rolled, or waved regardless of the length of hair cut on the rest of the head. However, this is not a hard and fast rule. Discuss your plans with your hairstylist to determine if the extra length on top is necessary for your basic styling needs.

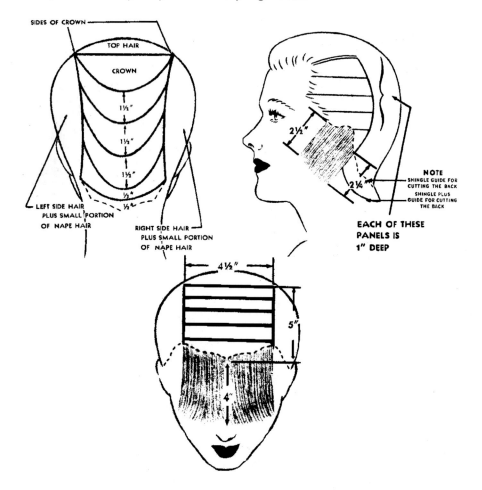

THE SHINGLE PLUS
SERVICEABLE SHORT

This is longer version of the shingle haircut found on the previous page. This cut is a great length for those that are trying to recreate wartime styles. The hair is cut about 2 1/2 inches in length, perfect to fit snugly under a service woman's cap and off her collar. Depending on how it was styled, this cut can also work for a late 1940s look when the poodle look was the rage.

NOTE
If your hair is stick straight and you don't plan on curling or perming it in any way, this haircut is not for you. The haircut works best on women with naturally wavy or curly hair.

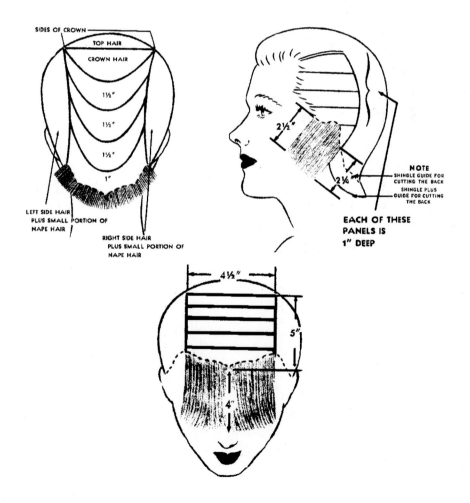

THE BABY
WAR TIME STANDARD

The hair is cut to three inches in length all around the head. This is my favorite length for wartime hairstyles. This haircut was very popular during the early 1940s and was considered fashionable on college campuses. Women were loping off their hair for the war effort but this length gave them much more flexibility with styling than the shorter cuts. When curled and styled, this haircut becomes curly around the ear area. This haircut is still considered rather short and was the standard length for women in the armed forces.

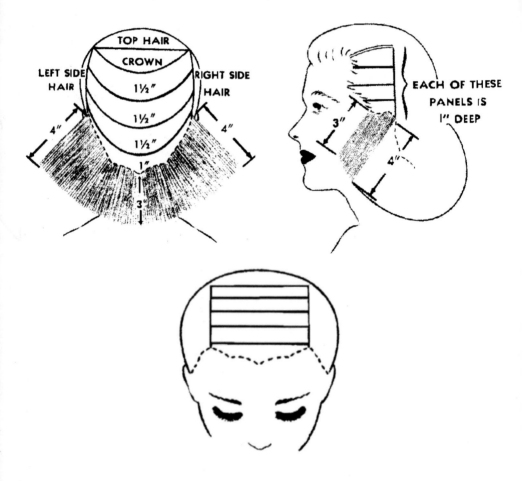

THE MIDDY
MOST POPULAR

A very versatile length, the hair is cut 4 inches long. This length became popular during the war with women who refused to cut their hair too short but still wanted to show support for the war effort. Considered a medium cut, this was the most popular length of the decade. It offered the most flexibility in styling techniques and could easily be worn up or down without much effort.

NOTE
Ivan of Hollywood was the first to introduce this haircut. It was considered the most flattering and ideal cut for most women of the period.

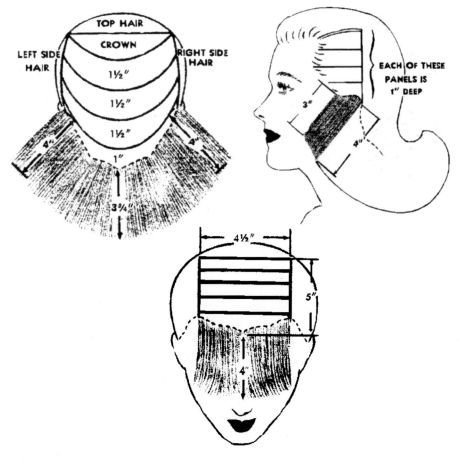

THE MIDDY PLUS
SCREEN SIREN

A very Hedy Lammarr length. The middy plus haircut is cut to about 4 1/2 inches in length and extends to the shoulder area. This cut lends itself very nicely to a smooth pageboy or curled fluff around the neck and shoulder area. This is also a convenient length for updos.

NOTE
All of the previous cuts have a slight curve to them, but here we begin to see the elongated "u" shape.

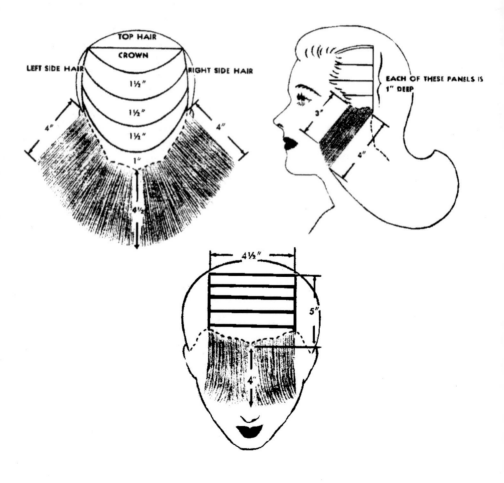

LONG LENGTH
FEMME FATALE

The is the length donned by various starlets including Rita Hayworth and Lana Turner. The length of this cut is 6 inches and comes to just below the shoulder area. This does not mean you have to cut your hair this short to insure a period look. If you'd like it longer, make sure to tell you stylist. A longer length is fine, but make sure not to lose the elongated "U" shape very apparent in the cut.

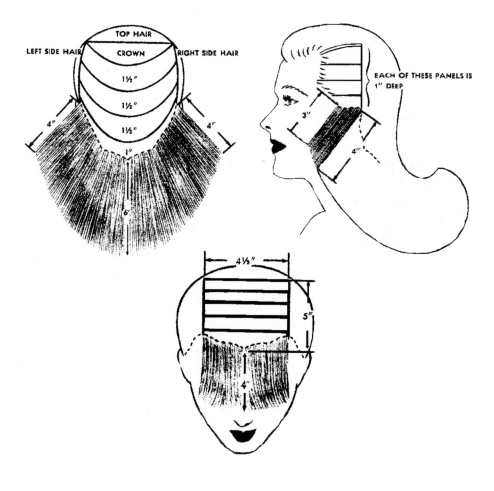

COMBINATION HAIRCUTS

Combination haircuts are just that - a combination of different lengths in order to get the look you want. The top hair, which is normally left 4-6 inches in length can be varied with any haircut depending on what your styling plans are. These cuts become very useful if you need extra length for rolls, waves, and pompadours. Any of the following cuts can be combined with any of the basic haircuts. Mix and match to create your own style and get the look you want.

TOP HAIR VARIATIONS

TOP REVERSE-ROLL LENGTH
The top hair near the face should be cut six inches in length and work its way back until it is five inches long, near the crown.

TOP HALF-WAVE REVERSE ROLL LENGTH
The top hair near the face should be cut six and one-half inches in length and work your way back until it is five and one-half inches long, near the crown.

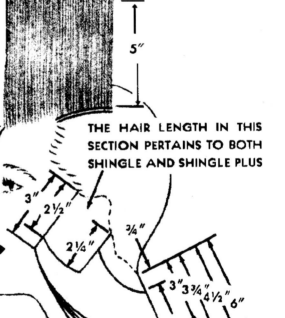

THE HAIR LENGTH IN THIS SECTION PERTAINS TO BOTH SHINGLE AND SHINGLE PLUS

TOP FULL WAVE REVERSE ROLL LENGTH
The top hair near the face should be cut seven inches in length and work your way back until it is six inches long, near the crown.

POMPADOUR LENGTH
The top hair near the face should be cut eight inches in length and work your way back until it is seven inches long, near the crown.

TOP HALF-WAVE POMPADOUR LENGTH

The top hair near the face should be cut eight and one-half inches in length and work your way back until it is seven and one-half inches long, near the crown.

TOP FULL WAVE POMPADOUR LENGTH

The top hair near the face should be cut nine inches in length and work your way back until it is eight inches long, near the crown.

SIDE HAIR VARIATIONS

SIDE REVERSE ROLL LENGTH

The hair nearest the face should be cut six inches in length and worked back until it's five inches in length.

SIDE HALF-WAVE REVERSE ROLL LENGTH

The hair nearest the face should be cut six and one-half inches in length and worked back until it's five and one-half inches in length.

SIDE FULL WAVE REVERSE ROLL LENGTH

The hair nearest the face should be cut seven inches in length and worked back until it's six inches in length.

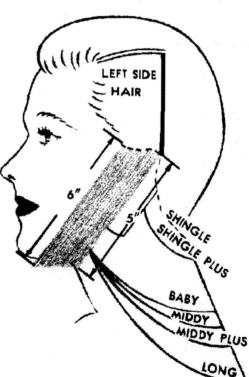

LEFT SIDE HAIR

6"

5"

SHINGLE
SHINGLE PLUS
BABY
MIDDY
MIDDY PLUS
LONG

CHAPTER TWO

THE BASICS

THE BASICS
HAIRSTYLE ELEMENTS, TERMS, AND
HOW-TOs

1940s hairstyles are made up of various elements that fit together to create a complete look. Before creating any 1940s hairstyle, you should understand what makes up a period do and how it is constructed. The techniques offered in this chapter, including both period and modern methods, and will allow you to recreate any of the styles shown in the remainder of this book.

You should be aware of the following terms, as they will be used extensively throughout the book:

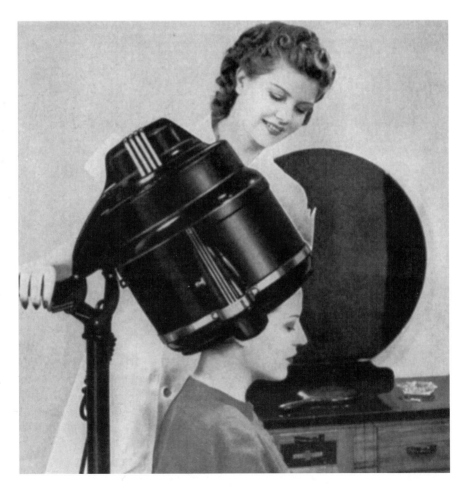

Backcomb – Holding the sectioned off hair away from head with one hand, comb the hair back towards the scalp while still holding the hair with the other hand. Only the backside of the section should be backcombed. The front (or part that will be facing outside) should be left as smooth as possible.

Barrel Curls – Curls that look like a hollow tube. Created by curling the hair with a curling iron and not combing the hair out afterwards.

Brush Out – After the curls have been set and dried, they are brushed out. Rolls, bangs, and pompadours should be brushed out separately.

Fluff – Fluff is the backbone behind most 1940s hairstyles. Brush the hair out to fluff it. Once the hair has been brushed a bit stick the brush towards the bottom of the hair and lift up, letting hair fall from the brush to create a fluffy mass.

Fluff Roll – A roll made of sectioned-off large barrel curls.

Hairspray – There are two types of hairsprays called for in this book. The first is a light hold hairspray that is used when curling the hair with a curling iron. The second is a medium hold hairspray that is used to spray the entire coiffure once it has been styled. Please make sure to only use a minimum amount to hold the hair, steering clear of creating a helmet head. For extra hold while dancing, parading, or picnicking, secure elements like rolls or pompadours in place by spraying the base of the element first. Once the base has been sprayed, blow-dry the base to harden the spray.

Loose Curls – Large curls that are used to just bend the hair instead of adding tons of curl. They are usually used to obtain smoother styles.

Pin Curls – Winding a one-half inch section of hair around your finger and then pinning in place to dry.

Ringlet Curls – Elongated tube shaped curls.

Sausage Curls – Small, tight barrel curls.

Smooth – To brush out curled hair vigorously to create a smoothed look to the curls. There should be no separate defined curl. All curls are brushed smooth. This styling creates volume, wave, and body without having the hair look curly.

Tight Curls – Very small curls with a small hollow center.

CURLS
SEE APPENDIX A FOR CURLING SUPPLIES

Very rarely did anyone in the 1940s have straight hair. If it wasn't naturally wavy or curly, you either had it permed and set, or curled it. That's just the way it was. If you had straight hair and did not want to have it permed and set (or had naturally wavy or curly hair and wanted it more manageable) you did one of the following:

CURLING METHODS
PIN CURLS
METHOD 1

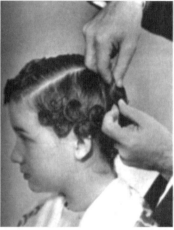

Start off with slightly damp hair and apply a setting lotion sparingly. Section off a piece of hair about half an inch wide. If too little hair is taken, the resulting curl will look frizzy, if too much hair is taken, the resulting curl will be flat. Half way up the section, place it on your index finger. Stretching it, wrap it smoothly around your finger. If you've wrapped it too tightly, you will notice having a hard time pulling the curl off of your finger. As you pull the ringlet off your finger, let the hollow circle in the center of the loop tighten. Once the loop has tightened a bit, roll the curl down to the base of the scalp and pin in place. Section off a new piece of hair, trying to keep each new section the same size as the last, until you've complete your full head or the section you want curled.

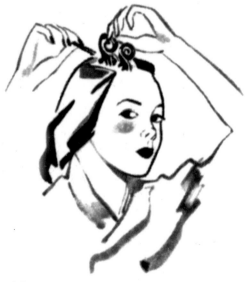

Pin curls created on the top of the head should be allowed to stand up while being secured by two bobby pins (or pin curl clips) intersecting in the hollow center of the curl. Pin curls created on the back of the head and on the sides should be allowed to lie flat while being secured by two bobby pins (or pin curl clips)

intersecting over the hollow center of the curl.

METHOD 2
Wind the curl starting at the base and working out. Tuck the ends into the center of the curl. Secure using two bobby pins (or pin curl clips) intersecting over the hollow center of the curl.

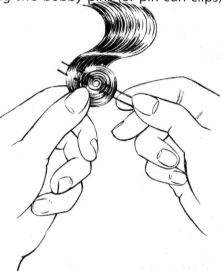

IMPORTANT NOTE
Make sure that when winding the curl in either method, you do not twist the section of hair. If the hair is twisted, the curls will not go in the direction you want them to.

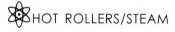HOT ROLLERS/STEAM ROLLERS
If you don't have time to pin curl or use regular curlers, hot rollers or steam rollers can be used to quickly curl the entire head of hair. Curls made in this way usually don't stay in as long as if they were pin curled, but hot rollers are a great quick fix if you're short on time.

CURLERS
Curlers come in a variety of sizes. Again, start with damp hair with added setting lotion. Use small curlers for tight curls and fluff, medium curlers for normal curls, and large curlers for extra body and wave.

PAPER CURLERS
Start off with a plain 8 ½ x 11 sheet of paper. Each sheet of paper will yield 4 curlers. Fold in half (top meets bottom) and then fold in half again. Unfold to reveal four equal sized pieces. Cut along the creases to create four separate strips of paper. Each paper strip should be approximately 2 ¾ inches wide and 8 ½ inches long. Roll up each paper strip making sure to end up with a 2 ¾ inch wide roll with a hollow center. Take a 1-inch section of hair; wrap it around the paper halfway down the section of hair. Roll the rest of the way down to the scalp. To secure the paper rolls in place pin each end with a bobbie pin making sure that one end of the bobbie pin goes through the hollow center of the curler and the other end into the hair on your scalp.

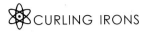CURLING IRONS

Curling irons can be used to create curls quickly. In order for the curling iron to work effectively, you'll need a light hold hairspray. Grasp a small section of hair and lightly spray it with a light hold hairspray. Roll it up in the curling iron and hear it sizzle. After holding it for a few more seconds, take the hair out of the curling iron. Let the hair sections cool down completely before attempting to brush them out. If you have a little extra time to spend, I recommend curling your hair with any of the previously mentioned methods. You will not only get a superior curl, but the curl will stay in the hair longer.

Curling irons come in different barrel widths. Here's a breakdown of different barrel widths and what their uses are:
Skinny – Tight pin curl like curls. Can be used to create small sections of pin curl wisps around the face. Also great for creating Betty Grable bangs depending on the length of hair. See our Bangs section for instructions.
Medium – Regular sized curls. Use this curling iron to curl hair instead of using the pin curl sets offered in the book. Unless otherwise noted, you can substitute all small area pin curl sets with a medium barreled curling iron.
Fat – Fat curls. The fat curling iron should really only be used to curl hair under in "pageboy" fashion.

RAG CURLERS
METHOD 1
Cut a bunch of 12-inch long strips of cotton fabric about an inch wide. Fold each strip in half to provide a thicker base for the hair to curl over. Take a 1-inch section of hair; wrap it around the fabric halfway down the section of hair. Roll the rest of the way down to the scalp and tie the ends of the fabric strip together to keep it in place.

METHOD 2
Cut a bunch of 6-inch long strips of fabric. Instead of the fabric folding in on itself to create support, wrap 2x4-inch long strips of magazine paper around the center portion of the fabric strip. Take a 1-inch section of hair; wrap it around the paper-wrapped fabric halfway down the section of hair. Roll the rest of the way down to the scalp and tie the ends of the fabric strip together to keep it in place.

PIPE CLEANER CURLERS

Pipe cleaners were and can be used exactly like the rag curlers, but instead of tying the ends together you twist them together. Now depending on the width of the pipe cleaner, you'll probably end up with some pretty tight curls. Unless your goal is to end up with a frizzy mess, I would recommend wrapping the hair around rather loosely.

From Rags to Curls, Circa 1945
Date tonight? Hair looking a little dim? Why don't you rag it?
It's a good trick suggested by the clever hair stylist, Lura de Gez, who believes in self-service. You can rag while you shower and dress. All you need are a few strips of clean cotton cloth about six by one and a half inches. Brush you r hair vigorously, divide it into sections, roll up each section on a rag and tie securely. Be careful to get all the little ends and to roll flat. For a pageboy make one row of curls (about eight). For fluffy ends, make two rolls of curls with less hair in each curl. Now take your shower. Be careful to keep your head away from the water; the damp warm air is all you need to set your hair. Leave the rags in while you dress and put on your lipstick. They lay a clean towel around your shoulders; unroll the rags and brush out the curls into smooth shining loveliness. It works!

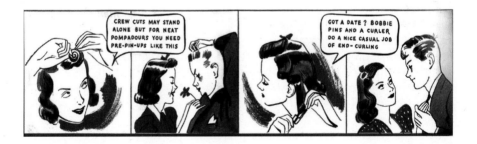

BASIC WAVES

Waves during the 1940s were deep and gently sloping. They were set into the hair permanently with pin curl sets at the beauty salon. Once the waves were set in the hair with a permanent, they could easily be combed in and replicated at home with a minimum of effort. When set properly, waves succeeded in adding interesting variations to otherwise simple styles.

There are very few beauticians, if any, that still practice permanently setting the hair to create waves. So, we've listed some alternative methods that you'll be able to try at home to get the same effect.

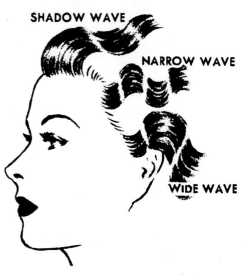

SHADOW WAVE

NARROW WAVE

WIDE WAVE

SHADOW WAVE
Shadow waves are wide and the ridges are not sharp. This type of wave looks very natural so you don't seem too made-up.

NARROW WAVE
The ridges of the narrow wave are sharp and close together. Do not use this wave unless you're going for a 1930s look.

HALF-WAVE
Half-waves are used to create a bit of height and movement to the hair, and are called for extensively throughout the sample styles section. It only means that instead of pulling the hair straight back, you create one ridge instead of two to add some interest. With any waving method you decide to use, make sure to brush the waves out thoroughly so they look deep and natural.

METHODS FOR CREATING WAVES

METHOD 1 - COMBING THEM IN
NOTE: Combing in waves is best suited for wavy or permed hair. It is very difficult to achieve good results using this method on straight hair. This method is not easy and does take practice and getting used to.

Starting with clean damp hair, add a setting lotion or light hold gel. Create your hair part. All waves should be constructed to match up

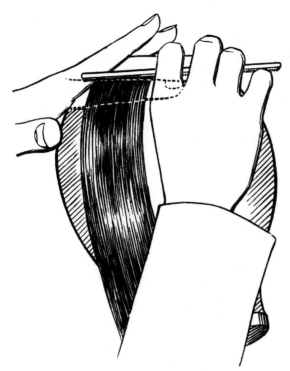

perpendicular to the part. (Disregard if you're trying to make a vertical wave.) Take a straight comb and hold it in the right hand (unless you're left handed) with three fingers at the top and the thumb and little finger underneath. See illustration. The left hand, as in the illustration (or your right if you're a lefty), holds the hair in place. Make sure that your left elbow is parallel with your left hand to ensure a tight grip.

Place the comb into the hair at a 90-degree angle between the index and middle finger of the left hand. Don't put too much weight on the comb, all is needed is for the comb to penetrate the hair down to the scalp. If the comb does not penetrate the hair down to the scalp, the resulting waves will look shoddy.

To create the first wave, move the comb in a semi-circleish direction to the right. See illustration. The comb should be kept in a straight position the entire time and parallel to your left index finger.

Once the first wave is completed, it is held down with the middle finger of the left hand. Moving the comb in a semi-circleish direction to the left creates the next wave. Continue down the head until you reach the end. If trying to create a vertical wave, the comb shouldbe perpendicular to the floor.

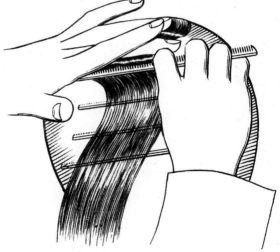

METHOD 2 - PIN CURLING

In order for the pin-curl method to work, you must be comfortable creating clean, tight pin curls.

Start by adding a setting lotion to clean, damp hair. Start a row of pin curls parallel to the direction you would like the waves to go (vertical or horizontal). If you'd like horizontal waves, start at the top and create a row of pin curls curling in a downward direction. The next row of pin curls should be created to curl in an upward direction. The third row should curl in a downward direction. The rows of pin curls should alternate until you've reached the end.

Once the pin curls have dried (make sure they are very, very dry), brush out the curls. Keep brushing until the curls turn into waves. To help this along, push the waves into place and spray with a light hairspray once waves are set. Vertical waves may also be achieved by alternating direction of pin curl rows.

See the Pin Curl Section for more information on how to create pin curls.

METHOD 3 - MODERN WAVING IRON

I have straight hair with absolutely no wave to it. I've tried the previous two methods on my hair, and they've failed miserably. That's not to say that they will not work on your hair, but I just don't have the magic touch needed to create waves. My method of waving requires a little cash, clean hair, a free bathroom, and an outlet.

One day, I overheard someone mention that there was an actual waving iron out on the market that could create waves in a matter of seconds instead of hours. Well, I went right out to my local beauty supply store and shelled out the $50.00 (Yes it is a hefty price) for a professional style "Marcel Waving Iron."

Here is what I discovered:
First off the waving iron has two settings, high and low. Since it is a professional strength tool, it gets very, very hot even on the low setting. It's also a little uncomfortable to use. The way it's supposed to be held takes some getting used to.

I tried both settings out to see what the difference was and what could be done with it. Basically the lower setting will give your hair a slight wave that is reminiscent of 1940s glamour waves. The higher setting will give your hair a tighter wave more along the lines of a 1930s Marcel wave (hence the name).

Unless you are going for a 1930s look, I recommend that you use the waving iron at a low setting on pieces of hair and not your whole head of hair. Use it to create waves in your side or top hair before you roll them into reverse rolls. You should not use the waving iron to do your whole head of hair (unless, again you're going for that 1930s look). It only tends to look messy and fried. If you want a full head of waves the previous two suggestions are still the way to go.

HAIR PARTS

The way your hair is parted in a period style will either make or break the look you're trying to go for. The goal is to find the most complementary hair arrangement that will end up making you look fabulous. The way you part your hair plays a major function in that goal.

COWLICK PART
Locate the point on your head where all of your hair seems to grow from. Once you've found that little point, make sure to comb all of your hair away from it. This part will give you a flat crown with a wheel of fluff around it. This is a great part that can be used when wearing a hat on the back portion of the head. It's also a fun part to be used with a really curly baby haircut. See Right.

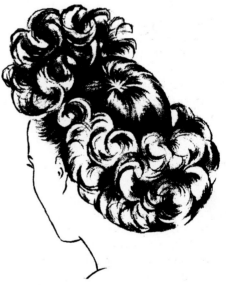

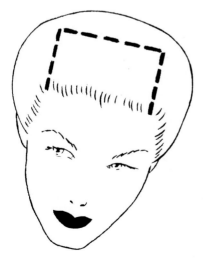

RECTANGULAR
A square part used to section off the hair for rolls, pompadours, or bangs. See Left.

21

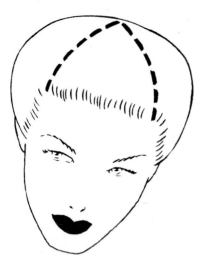

V

A "V" shaped part used to section off the hair for rolls, pompadours, or bangs. Use this part if you're going for "Betty Page" bangs. See Left.

EAR TO EAR

This part is a way to section off the front hair from the back hair. This part can be used when creating an up-do.

Sectioning the hair off in this way makes it very easy to roll the front and pin up the back without creating a messy coiffure. See Right.

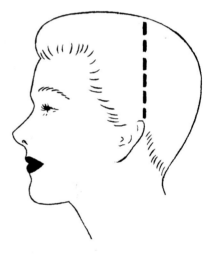

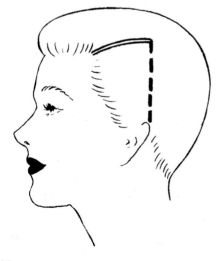

CROWN TO EAR

This part is basically used to section off hair for side styles like waves or rolls. See Left.

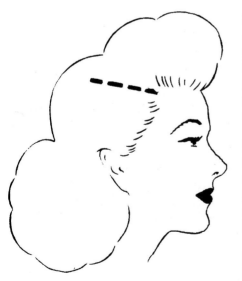

BACK DIAGONAL
The back diagonal part was very popular in France from 1938-1939. The style then migrated to the Untied States in the early 1940s. This is a great part for adding back interest to an up-do, but keeping it looking clean make take more practice than you think.

VARIATION
Another part for adding back interest to an up-do is to create a part down the center of the back. This makes it easy to roll the sectioned pieces toward or away from each other. Again, another one that's difficult to keep clean.

SIDE
A side part was and still is the most popular way to part the hair. The slight variation of curving the side part upward will add a more glamorous overtone to the coiffure.

DIAGONAL SIDE
Make the side part slightly diagonal. This is a great method to place more hair on the smaller side, great for women with thin hair.

NOTE
Place the palm of your hand on the crown of your head and press forward. This will make the hair break into a natural part.

ROLLS

Rolls are what make a 1940s hairstyle look like a 1940s hairstyle. They can be considered a staple ingredient in the process of constructing a period looking hairstyle. The rolls of the 1940s were medium sized and soft. For those of us with thick or medium weight hair, these are fairly easy to accomplish using curling and backcombing. For those that cringe at the idea of backcombing, or for those who have thin hair, don't fret; there is a solution.

THE OLD WAY
Pin curls, pin curls, pin curls.
If you'd like to this the authentic way, you need pin curls, setting lotion, hairspray, a comb, and a tough scalp that can take a beating.
Apply setting lotion to damp hair and set with pin curls. Setting diagrams are included within the chapter.
When dry, comb out the curl. Depending on how thick your hair is, you may just be able to roll the hair and pin it. If your hair needs more volume, backcombing is the answer. On the underside (the part of the hair that will not be facing the outside world) of the section of hair you'd like to roll, backcomb the hair slightly (holding the hair away from head with one hand, comb the hair back towards the scalp while still holding with the other hand) to give yourself volume to roll the hair over. Smooth the outside of the section a bit before rolling, making sure not to loose any of the volume you've just created. Smooth the hair over the palm of your hand, tuck the ends under and pin securely.

CURLING IRON METHOD

A curling iron can come in handy if you need to create rolls in a hurry. Grasp a small section of hair and lightly spray it with a light hold hairspray. Roll it up in the curling iron and hear it sizzle. After holding it for a few seconds, take the hair out of the curling iron. Let each section of hair cool down completely before attempting to brush it out. Once the hair sections have cooled down, you can backcomb, roll, and secure.

RATS!
Stockings
During the first half of the twentieth century, a woman would save the hair that had accumulated in her hairbrush. Once there was enough hair gathered, she would stuff a stocking full of it and use it to roll her hair over for increased volume. This method can be recreated today.

⚛ MODERN RATS - FOAM DOUGHNUTS

(Thank you to Lora Boehm - Hairstylist Extraordinaire, for this great idea)
Take a trip to your local beauty supply store and find those foam doughnuts that are used to create buns and chignons. These synthetic wonders can be used for a number of styling purposes. How they work is simple. Each doughnut is made of a stiff, foamy material. Hair is wrapped over and around the foamy material to create volume. To secure the foam section in place you will need metal bobbie pins. Since modern bobbie pins come with rubber tips, you'll need to bite off one rubber tip from each bobbie pin. The sharp side (the side without the rubber tip) is inserted into the stiff foam section, while the scalp friendly rubberized side is inserted into the hair. Buy a few doughnuts so that you can use them in the following ways:

1. "As is" to create a bun or chignon
2. Cut through one side so you are left with one single long tube. This can be used for a continuous roll around the back or front.
3. Cut the doughnut into sections that hair can be rolled over.

SPECIAL NOTE
Make sure that you taper down the ends of any cut foam piece. They'll be easier to cover and will mold to the shape of your head more naturally. Also: please, please, please make sure to cover up each foam piece completely. There is nothing worse than exposing the secrets of your fabulous do.

The following diagrams are explained using pin curl sets. Hair should be set in numbered order so you can achieve the correct effect. However, you can substitute the pin curl sets with whatever curling method you like.

TOP ROLLS

Almost all top rolls start out with a rectangular part. Remember, the more hair you use to create the roll, the thicker and more solid the roll will become. If creating rolls with pin curls, remember that the pin curls should be set standing up.

TOP REVERSE ROLL
The most common roll found in 1940s hairstyles. All other top rolls are modifications and variations on this basic roll.

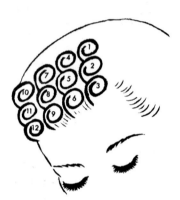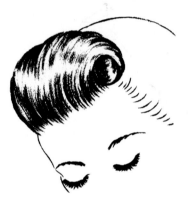

TOP HALF-WAVE REVERSE ROLL
In order to achieve this effect, create a half wave before curling the rest of the hair. Two rows of pin curls are standard for this type of roll. If you'd like a larger roll, add a third row of pin curls. See Diagram Below.

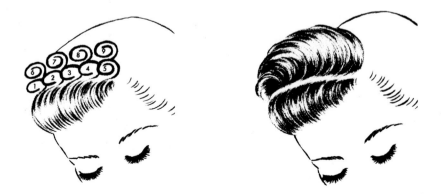

TOP FULL WAVE REVERSE ROLL
This is a very soft and elegant set. The diagram shows how to create this wave using a pin curl method. This look can also be created with a waving iron, and ends curled under with a curling iron. See Diagram Below.

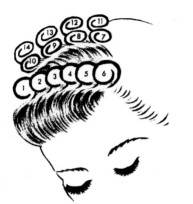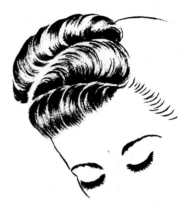

SIDE ROLLS

Basic side rolls add lift, interest, and volume to any 1940s hairstyle. Instead of pinning the sides straight back, add some interest by adding rolls and waves.

SIDE REVERSE ROLL
The side reverse roll, like the top reverse roll, is pretty much a staple in 1940s hairstyles. All other side rolls are modifications and variations on this basic roll. See Diagram Below.

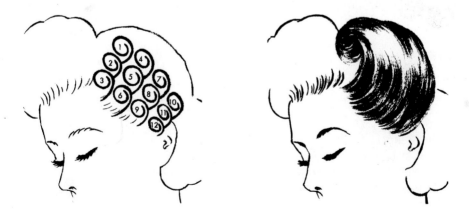

SIDE HALF-WAVE REVERSE ROLL

To create this look a half wave must be made in the side hair before the ends are curled. Combing the hair up first and then shaping it will give it a very beautiful, flowing effect. See Diagram Below.

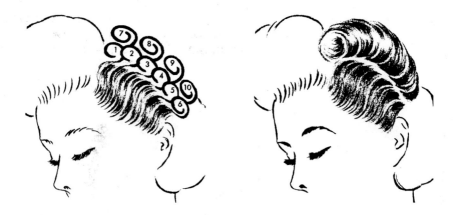

SIDE FULL WAVE REVERSE ROLL

The diagram pictured, shows how to create the wave using a pin curl set. This look can also be created with a waving iron, and ends curled under with a curling iron. See Diagram Below.

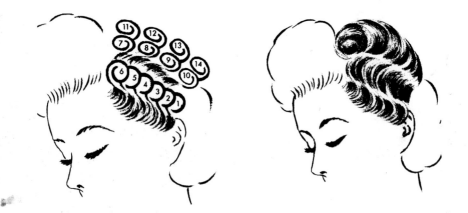

OTHER ROLL VARIATIONS

Without changing the pin curl settings, each roll previously listed, can be modified by combing the hair forward instead of back. Combing the hair forward will create a forward roll (a fun variation from the normal reverse roll).

POMPADOURS

There are three basic pompadour settings, each a variation of the next. The setting instructions for pompadours are exactly the same as for rolls only longer hair is used. To get a true pompadour the hair must stand pretty high. This requires a lot of backcombing so it can damage the hair if you use this style on a regular basis. Instead of backcombing, you can use rats to create volume without sacrificing quality.

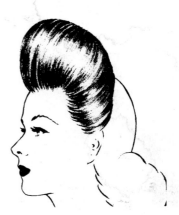

STRAIGHT BACK POMP
This is a much higher version of the top and side reverse rolls, and setting instructions are exactly the same. Set longer hair into a top reverse roll and side reverse rolls. When dry backcomb, or use a rat, smooth over the front, and roll over to create a nice, high, pomp.

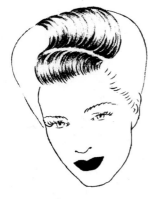

HALF-WAVE POMP
This look is a higher version of the top half-wave reverse roll. Set the hair the same way you would for a top half-wave reverse roll and side half wave reverse rolls. The half-wave in the pomp creates a softness that was more popular than the straight back pomp during the 1940s. When dry, either backcomb or use a rat, smooth over the front, and roll over to create a nice, high, pomp. Before pinning in place make sure to push the wave into form.

FULL WAVE POMP

Full wave pomps are glamour to the extreme. The hair is set the same way as for the top full wave reverse roll and the side full wave reverse rolls. Again, as in the side and top full wave reverse rolls, you can use a waving iron to create the waves and creases in the hair. When dry, either backcomb or use a rat, smooth over the front, and roll over to create a nice, high, pomp. Make sure to push the wave into form before pinning in place.

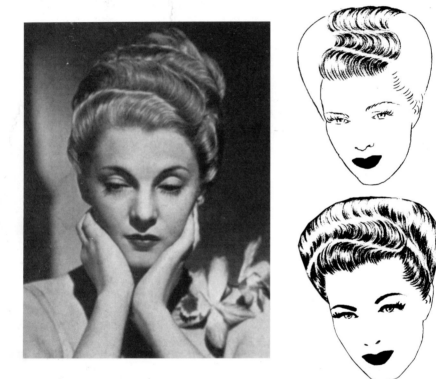

HOW TO KEEP YOUR POMP LOOKING FRESH

Women in the 1940s would generally get their hair set once a week. In between settings, they needed to find ways to keep the hairstyle looking fresh instead of flat. Here is a period tip on just how to do that:

First you should comb out the entire pompadour. Then part the hair neatly. Make sure that the part is curved in a half-moon shape (with the curve towards the back of the head), and that it ends an inch above the ears. This is to ensure that when the hair is set, the part will not be seen. Comb the topknot forward, shape it over your hand, and push into place. Comb the sides back up. If the roll is flat or limp, tease the hair a little. Tuck the sides underneath the topknot and mold into a smooth pompadour.

BANGS

Bangs are a great way to camouflage imperfections and to add interest to period hairstyles. There are six basic bang shapes that were popular during the 1940s. Of course any of the bang shapes can be modified to create an original look all your own.

FORWARD ROLL BANGS

The hair for these bangs should be five inches long in front and seven inches long in back. Making a rectangular part, set the hair as you would for a top reverse roll or curl with a curling iron. When the set has dried, or the hair has cooled (if using a curling iron), brush out the curls, roll forward over the palm of the hand (tucking the ends under), and pin securely.

BETTY GRABLE BANGS

For Betty Grable bangs you need bangs that are three to four inches in length. If they're shorter, they'll frizz, if they're longer the curls will be too large. Section off your bangs by using a rectangular part. Set the hair as shown, or use a skinny barrel curling iron to create the tight curls needed. If using a skinny barrel curling iron, make sure that you section off each curl as in the illustration. When the set has dried, or the hair has cooled (if using a curling iron), brush out the curls and fluff. These are great bangs to use with any curly up-do.

HALF-WAVE BANGS

The hair for these bangs should be four inches long in front and six inches long in back. Making a rectangular part, set the hair as in the illustration, or curl with a curling iron (making sure to curl the first row away from the face). When the set has dried, or the hair has cooled (if using a curling iron), brush out the curls, and push the half-wave into place. See Diagram Below.

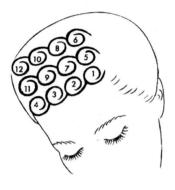
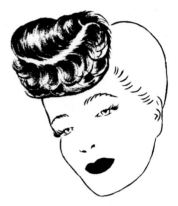

FULL WAVE BANGS

The hair for these bangs should be five and a half inches long in front and seven and a half inches long in back. Making a rectangular part, set the hair as in the illustration or else wave with a waving iron (making sure to curl the ends with a curling iron). When the set has dried, or the hair has cooled (if using the iron), brush out the curls and push the full wave into place. See Diagram Below.

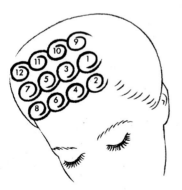
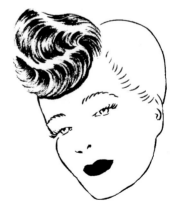

CHAPTER THREE

SELECTING THE RIGHT HAIRSTYLE

HOW TO MAKE SURE YOUR HAIR LOOKS FABULOUS

You need choose a hairstyle that will flatter your best features and camouflage your imperfections. This chapter will help you figure out what style will look best on you based on period Hollywood Studio Standards.

THE FIVE FACE TYPES

OVAL
People that have an oval shaped face are extremely lucky because any style will look good on them. See Diagram to Right.

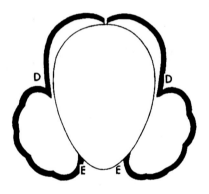

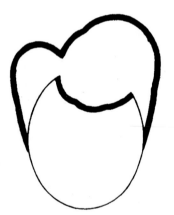

ROUND
The round face shape requires that the hairstyle you wear contain height to elongate the face. An up-do works great for this. See Diagram to Left.

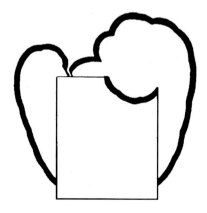

SQUARE
A square shaped face needs a hairstyle that will soften its angular lines. Fullness at the temples and/or jaw should do the trick. See Diagram to Right.

LONG

The long face needs a hairstyle that will make it appear shorter and more round. Fullness in the bang area and near the jaw line should work.

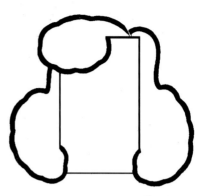

TRIANGLE/HEART

The triangle/heart shaped face also needs softness around its angular portions. Height at the top and fluff at the jaw line looks great. If you happen to have an upward triangle shape instead of a downward triangle shape, width needs to be added to the narrow temple area and subtracted from the wider jaw line.

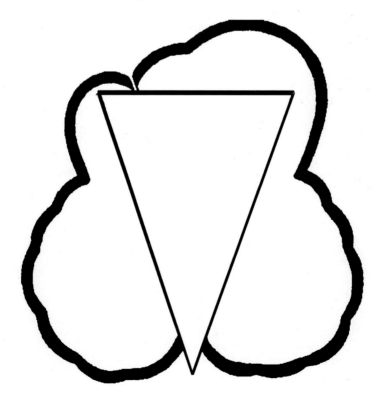

CAMOUFLAGE IMPERFECTIONS

Everyone has imperfections. The studio system that produced Hollywood screen sirens were masters at camouflaging flaws and making women look perfect. The following are some standard studio tricks that can be used to balance and hide imperfections.

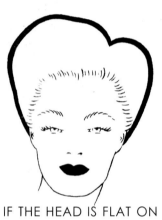

IF THE HEAD IS FLAT ON
TOP

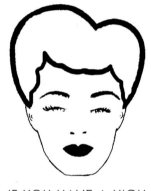

IF YOU HAVE A HIGH
FOREHEAD

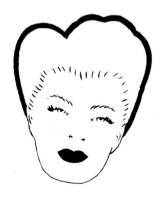

IF YOU HAVE A SHORT
FOREHEAD

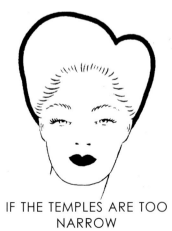

IF THE TEMPLES ARE TOO
NARROW

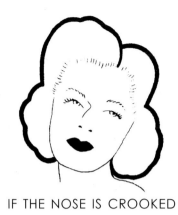

IF THE NOSE IS CROOKED

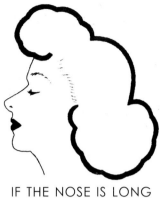

IF THE NOSE IS LONG

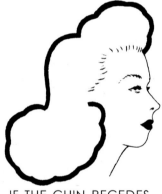

IF THE CHIN RECEDES

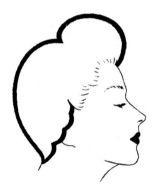

IF THE EARS ARE LARGE

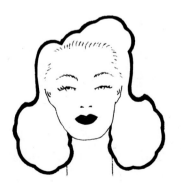

IF THE NECK IS TOO LONG

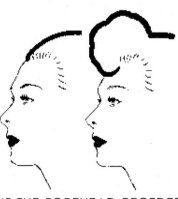

IF THE FOREHEAD RECEDES

HOLLYWOOD HOWDY – DOs, CIRCA 1946

The moving picture stars are just like you when it comes to their hairdos. Some of them, like you, love change and can be counted on to follow the latest hair fashions or to set new ones. Here are ten tips to help you figure out what style is best for you.

1. Type of Hair. Curly hair and strong healthy hair have body, which is a great help to a hairdo. Nowadays with permanent waves no one needs to have straight hair unless she thinks it's for her.

2. Amount of Hair. In general, heavy hair looks better in smooth flat arrangements; thin hair can stand more fluff.

3. Special Difficulties. Bangs will sometimes camouflage a poor forehead line and a bob haircut or a knot of hair may hide the less-than-good hairline at back of neck. Never try to force hair against the way that it grows. Changing a part often gets around a cowlick.

4. Your Skill. If your fingers are all thumbs, choose something simple. But you can probably learn!

5. Your Time. Better wear a style you can whip up neatly in the time available than to shuffle together something elaborate that may soon fall apart.

6. The Latest Style. It's good to be in fashion if the fashion is good for you. With a little ingenuity you can usually adapt a trying style so you look smart and pretty.

7. The Scene. Office hairdos in the office, party hairdos at the party. Enough said.

8. Your Clothes, especially hats. Lines of hairdo should have the right relation to the costume. In any hat versus hair controversy, either adapt your hairstyle or buy a different hat.

9. Your Poise. Perhaps most important. The best rule is: wear a hairdo which you feel is yours, one so pleasantly under control that you can forget it and avoid fiddling. You know what I mean!

TWELVE MUSTS FOR A GOOD HAIR-DO

1.   It does something for your face.

2.   It is practical for your kind of hair.

3.   It is well proportioned to your figure.

4.   It is right for your age.

5.   It shows proper respect for fashion.

6.   It looks neat and well groomed.

7.   It suits your way of living.

8.   It is equally good with or without your hat.

9.   It can be adapted to special social occasions.

10.   You can get the necessary professional care (cut or wave) in your neighborhood.

11.   You can keep it looking nice yourself between visits to the hairdresser.

12.   Your friend's often say, "How nice your hair looks."

CHAPTER FOUR
BASIC STYLES

CASUAL GAL

No matter what their age and no matter what their preference in hair styling is, the women of America have declared themselves emphatically on at least one point — their coiffures should be feminine and neat.

Yes, her very life, her home, the man she will marry, often depends on the art of bringing fresh loveliness to her hair. (Circa 1942)

CUTE STYLES FOR SHORT HAIR

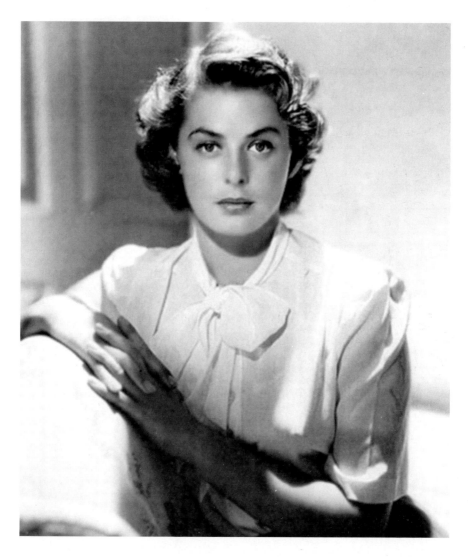

INGRED BERGMAN

Ingred Bergman's hair is about 3 1/2 - 4 inches long and layered in this photo. To reproduce this look, part the hair on the side and curl the side and back hair using pin curls, curlers, or hot rollers. The top hair closest to the forehead should be curled forward and under and the rest of the top hair should be curled away from the face. This is not a very curly do, so make sure that your curls are medium sized. When dry or cool, comb the hair out and style.

SKULLCAP COIFFURE, CIRCA 1942
This style has a smooth crown surrounded by short, soft brushed-out curls. The side hair is slightly waved away from the face and the bangs are brought slightly over the forehead.

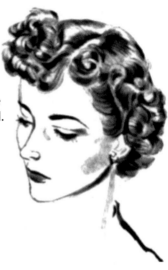

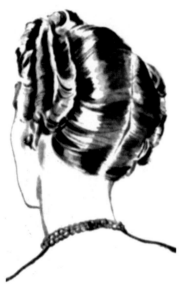

NEAT NECKLINE, CIRCA 1942
For the woman who wants a neat neckline and abhors the short cut look. This style uses a part from the side center front to center back. The front hair is waved softly and back hair is brushed smoothly from the part and held with small barrettes. This style also works nicely with gray hair.

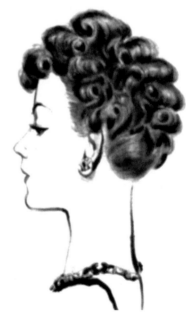

FLOWER PETAL, CIRCA 1942
The hair is cut short after it is set. Each row of curls is cut a different length so that when brushing, the curls fall naturally into a hairdo pattern like the petals of a flower.

UP OR DOWN FOR SHORT HAIR,
Circa 1943

Hair should be about three inches long and can be styled to go either up or down with this setting.

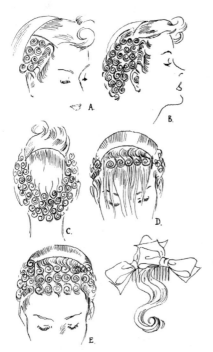

SETTING INSTRUCTIONS

1. Make an ear to ear part.

2. Wave the side hair and pin curl the ends.

3. Set the top hair in three rows of curls alternating directions.

4. Set the back hair in pin curls, keeping the crown flat and smooth.

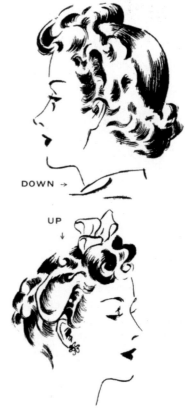

For the down style, simply fluff out the back and comb out the sides. Top hair should be brushed out and arranged in fluff curls. For the up style, simply comb the back hair in an upward direction and pin securely. Use a hairpiece attached to a comb to secure behind the top hair. This will add curl and coverage over the crown area.

SMOOTH MEDIUM LENGTH STYLES

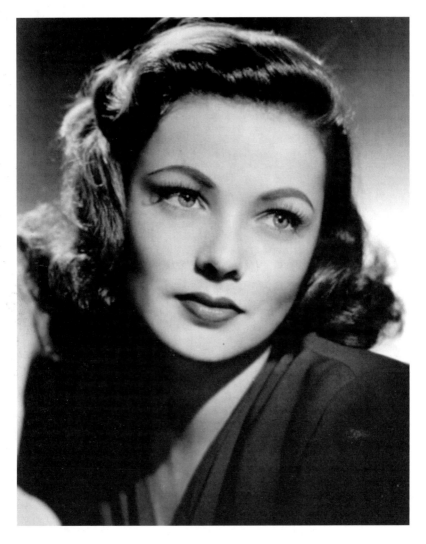

GENE TIERNEY

Gene Tierney's hair is a little above shoulder length and layered. Her top hair is cut 4-5 inches in length. To reproduce this style you should first part the hair on the side near the temple area. All the top hair is curled back and way from the face. The rest of the hair is curled. When dry or cool, brush the hair out vigorously, making sure to flip the ends outward. Tussle the hair a bit. The top hair should be combed back away from the face and the ends left to fall in a little curl near the temple opposite the part.

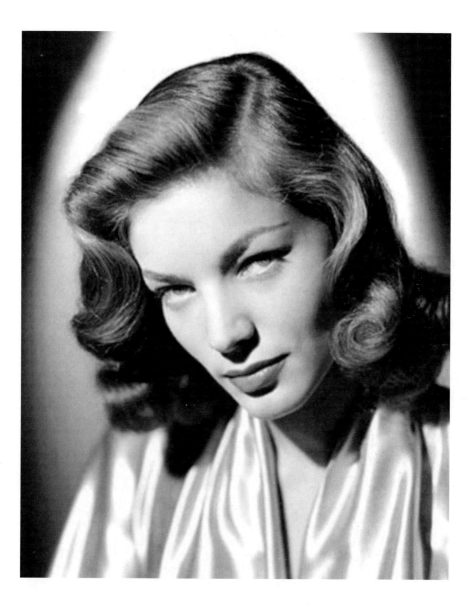

LAUREN BACALL

Lauren Bacall's hair is a little above shoulder length and slightly layered. The top hair is kept fairly long so that it can be waved. To reproduce this style you should first part the hair on the side. Curl all the top hair back and away from the face. The hair closest to the face on the sides is curled forward toward the face and the rest is curled away from the face. The back is set into loose curls. When hair is dry or cool, brush hair out until smooth , pushing the waves into place.

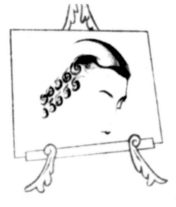

VARIATIONS ON A SET

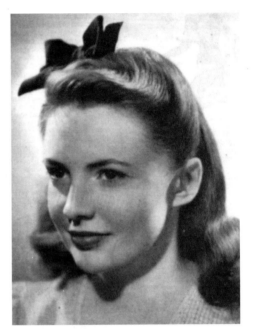

The hairstyles on these two pages can all be derived from the set shown above. For added appeal, half waves can be added to the top hair at the hairline to create bend and height.

For the hairstyles shown on this page, the hair is parted in the center or on the side, combed smooth, then pulled back and secured.

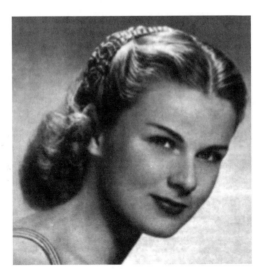

PAGEBOY

For a pageboy look, you can use the set as shown on the previous page. When the set is dry, comb the hair smooth and flip the ends under.

Again, half waves can be added to the side and top hair to add interest and bend.

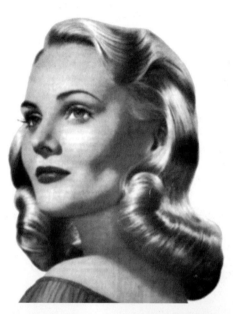

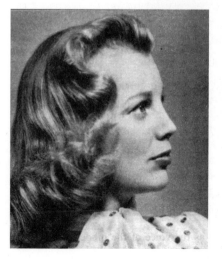

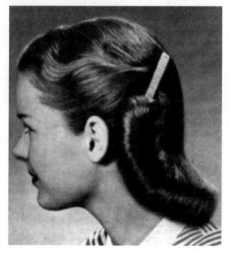

CURLY STYLES FOR MEDIUM HAIR

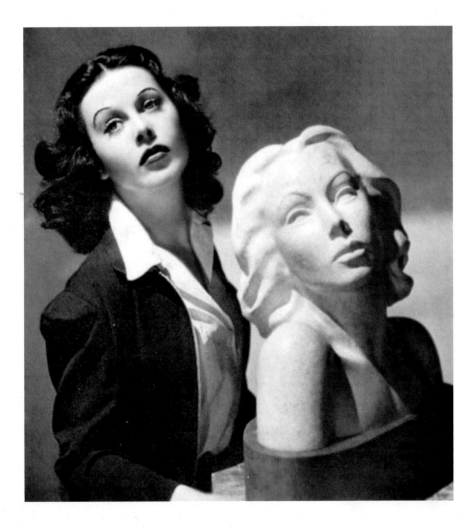

HEDY LAMMARR

Hedy Lammarr's hair is shoulder length and layered. To reproduce this look, part the hair down the center and curl the rest of the hair using pin curls, hot rollers, or curlers. When dry or cool, brush out the curls and fluff up a bit.

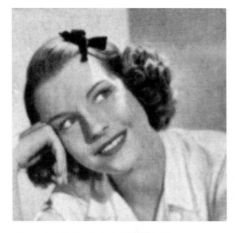

SIMPLE STYLE
Hair length should be just above shoulder length and layered. Part the hair to the side and pin curl the ends in two or three rows all around the head. When dry fluff out the ends and add a bow.

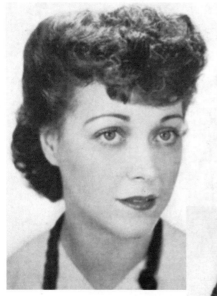

ROLLS AND FLUFF
Hair is about 4 inches long. Sides are set into reverse rolls and secured with combs.

The back hair ends are set into pin curls and then fluffed out a bit. Make sure to let the curls retain some of their tightness. The top hair is set into fluff bangs.

STYLES FOR LONGER HAIR

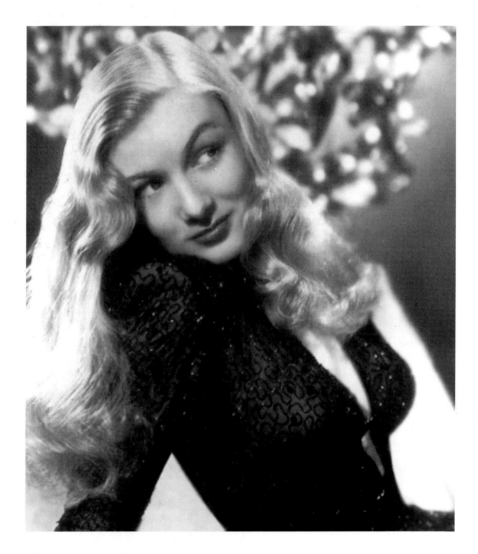

VERONICA LAKE
Veronica Lake's hair comes to the middle of her back and is slightly layered. To recreate her classic "peekaboo" bangs, you should start off with a side part. The top hair nearest the face is curled forward. The rest of the top hair is curled backward away from the face. The rest of her hair is slightly waved with the ends curled and fluffed.

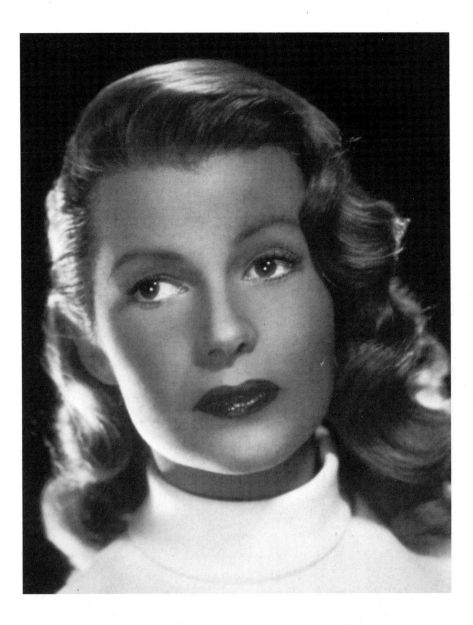

RITA HAYWORTH

Rita Hayworth's hair is a little below shoulder length and layered. To reproduce this look start with a center part. Create waves in the hair while keeping the top of the head and crown smooth. Please refer to the "Basic Elements" chapter for instructions on how to create waves. Once the waves have been created, brush the hair smooth. Pull back and secure the smaller side while letting the other side drop into smooth waves.

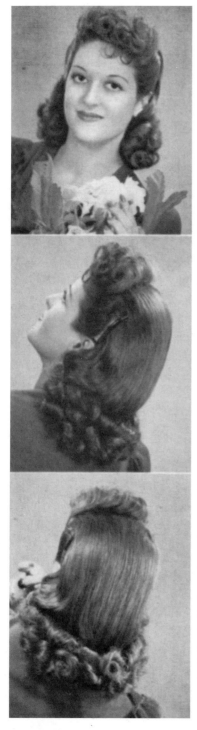

CURLS FOR
LONG HAIR

TIPS

1. Dampen the hair with water and only a small amount of setting lotion. This will save considerable drying time.
2. Roll the ends loosely as the curls must be soft. When doing the back, do not roll the pin curls above the nape of the neck.
3. Use combs at the sides to support the weight of the hair and to keep it from scattering over the ears. You can use plain combs for daytime wear or flowered, jeweled, or phosphorescent ones for evening allure.
4. Do not remove the combs when finishing the style, just comb through the hair above and below them.
5. When brushing out the hair, roll the hair lightly over your fingers, being careful to avoid any suggestion of a tight, sausage effect. The soft pompadour is merely brushed out, fringed bang is set in place and the rest falls in light, puffy ringlets.

SETTING INSTRUCTIONS
(shown on opposite page):

1. Start off with long hair.
2. Part the top hair using a V part and pin curl hair as show in photo.
3. Comb the hair on the sides up and back and secure with a comb. Pin curl ends of side hair going in an upward direction as shown in photograph.
4. Do the same on the other side.
5. Comb the back straight down and pin curl the ends in two rows going in an upward direction.

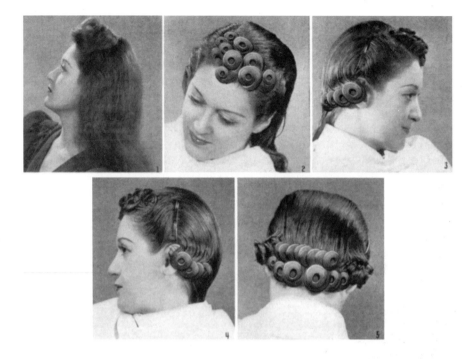

The hairstyle below is a variation on this basic set. The back hair would be set the same way and then combed out to form a nice full roll. The top and side hair would be set into modified full wave reverse rolls.

The hairstyle below is also a variation on this basic set. The back hair would be set going under instead of over and then combed into a page boy. The top hair is set into forward roll bangs and the sides are set into reverse rolls.

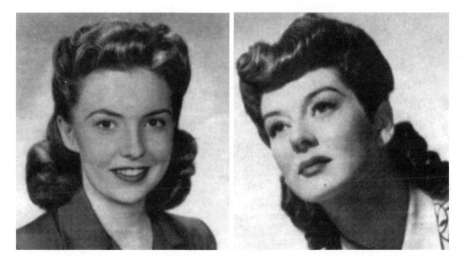

GREAT SUMMERTIME STYLE

For this style you need damp, almost dry hair. Make a center part and dampen the front hair with setting lotion. Mold into full waves on either side of the part. Set the hair above each ear into two large reverse rolls. The back hair is set with clockwise pin curls. When dry brush out the hair. Sweep the front and side sections up and back and secure with bobbie pins. Tie with a ribbon or handkerchief. Brush out back hair thoroughly until waves form. Let ends fall into natural curls.

VARIATIONS
Press the front hair into waves just like the previous version, but roll the back hair. If you want a more sophisticated clean look, omit the front waves and arrange the back into a narrow pageboy (smooth the back hair and curl the ends under).

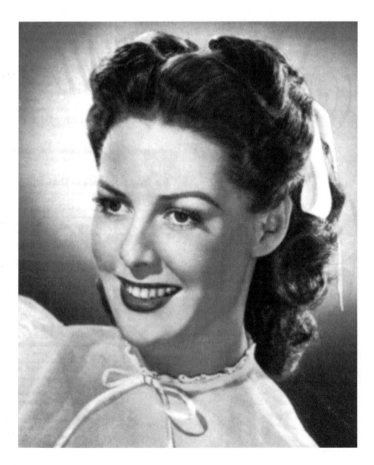

CONTINUOUS ROLL

Make an ear to ear part. Curl hair and create front and side reverse rolls. Smooth down the crown and make a continuous reverse roll along the nape.

TIP

Use a foam rat to roll the hair around. Secure with metal bobbie pins. See "Basic Elements" section on how to use rats for more information.

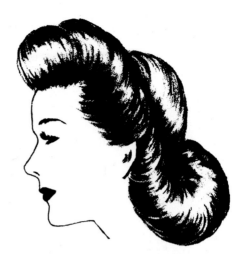

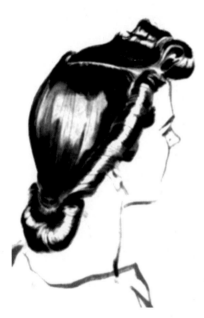

CONTINUOUS ROLL VARIATION

Create a forward roll for the top hair. Roll the side hair in to a continuous roll, meeting at the nape of the neck. Secure hair with a brooch and roll the ends under.

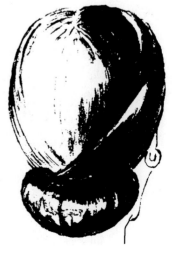

ROLL AT NAPE OF NECK

Make a center part and comb hair to the back. Criss-cross side hair at nape and secure with bobbie pins—two pointing up, two down. Make a solid roll, pin and add an invisible net around the roll. This is a good style for keeping long hair out of the way.

STYLES FOR WOMEN WHO WEAR GLASSES

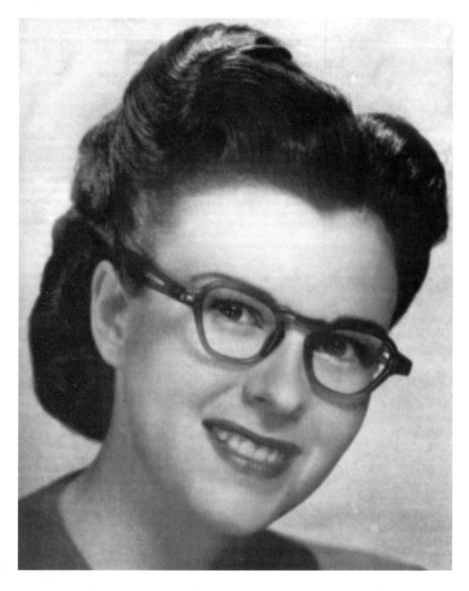

To recreate this style, start with the hair parted to the side. Create a half wave in the top hair and bring the sides up into reverse rolls. The back is curled and secured with a snood or hairnet.

UPSWEPT SIDES

Sweep up the sides and pin at the high part of the crown. Tie a bow. This will definitely give some added height and is very simple to do. You can pin curl the back hair to add some extra cuteness. Try to stay away from parting the hair down the center. A center part is usually not flattering for women who wear glasses.

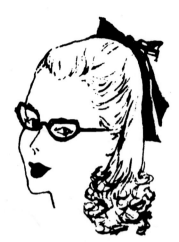

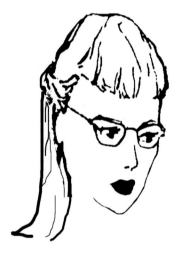

FLAT BANGS

If you have a long face and wear glasses, consider bangs cut flat to hide a long forehead. Glasses also look really great with bangs cut short.

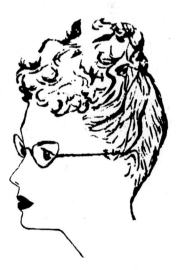

FLUFFY BANGS

Fluffy bangs give the needed height to a hairdo and make a pretty hairline. Pin curl the top and fluff out when dry. Sweep up the back hair in a flat roll and pin behind the fluff bangs.

CAREER GAL

Today every woman that's worth her salt is working some job. If she isn't working in a defense plant or an office, then she's devoting every free moment to volunteer work to help the war effort. She want to look feminine and attractive, but at the same time she wants to look smart and efficient on the job.

(Circa 1943)

SHORT HAIR WITH SOFT CURLS

Hair length should be 3 - 4 inches. The top hair is set in a half wave reverse roll. For the sides, first make a half wave then pin curl the ends. The back is set in many pin curls. When the hair dries, brush the curls out thoroughly.

You can get a smooth or curly looking depending on how you comb out the do.

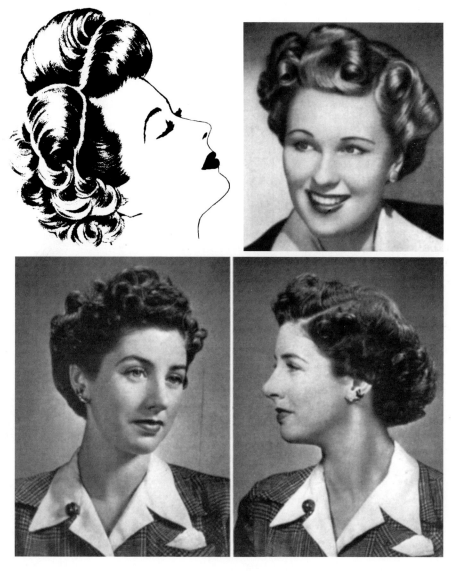

ADJUSTABLE HAIRDO

The hairstyle below is very adaptable and can be slightly modified to be proportionate to the shape of your face. The crown hair is smoothed down and the left side is brought up into a reverse roll. The right side is set into a modified wave reverse roll. The back hair is curled under and fanned to the sides in pageboy fashion.

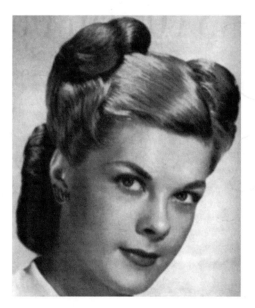

Below are examples of how this hairstyle can be adapted to different face types:

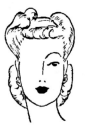

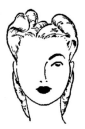

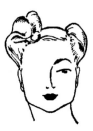

HIGH FOREHEAD   ROUND FACE   WIDE JAW

CAREER GIRL CLASSIC, Circa 1942

Hairstyle by Dumas

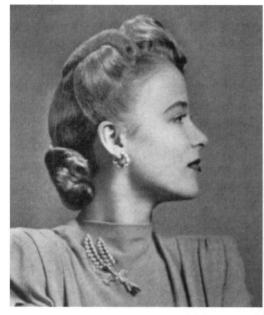

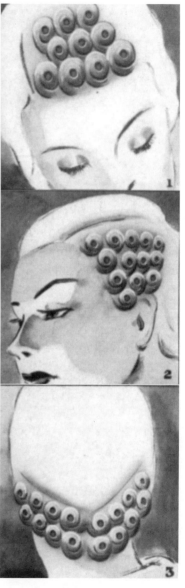

The style is simple and neat in appearance and though its smooth, trim lines leave no margin for intricate detail, it possesses an air that is casual and different. The hair is shorter which makes it easy and manageable between professional sets.

SETTING INSTRUCTIONS

1. The top section is set in diagonal rows of pin curls that stand up from the head.
2. On the left side the curls are set in diagonal rows with curls wound counterclockwise. The right side is set the same way except the curls are wound in a clockwise direction.
3. In back, the curls are set in a V formation and are wound up and toward the center of the head.

REQUISITION A NEW HAIRDO, Circa 1943

Hairstyle by Miriam Cordwell

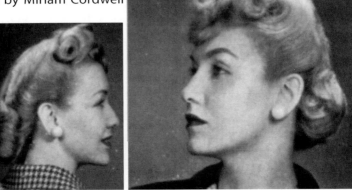

Well-turned waves that can be depended upon to look neat and trim at all times. This is a two-way style that can be combed in to a waved pomp for tailored suits or into soft bangs for a more casual style. Hairpins keep the upswept sides in line.

SETTING INSTRUCTIONS

1. The hair is parted on the left side and across the crown of the head. A small half-wave is formed at the forehead. Set two rows of curls in counter clockwise direction.

2. On the left side set two vertical rows of curls, the first winding counterclockwise, the second winding clockwise.

3. On the right side the hair is combed back into a vertical wave and all of the curls are wound clockwise

4. When dry, brush the hair smooth and style as in picture. For a more casual look, fluff the bangs forward.

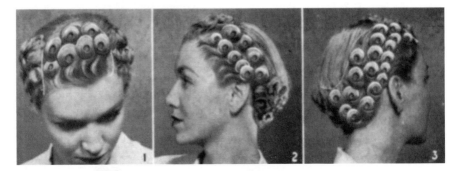

WORKING WAVES, Circa 1943

Hairstyle by Joseph Scherer

These waves, for both youthful beauty and practical handling, are made from both pin curls and waves. The parting of the style guides the general lines and adds an interesting touch to the back.

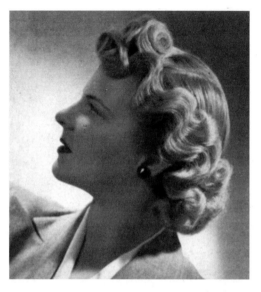

SETTING INSTRUCTIONS
1. The top hair is rolled into rows of pin curls alternating direction each row.
2. The side hair is combed back in two diagonal

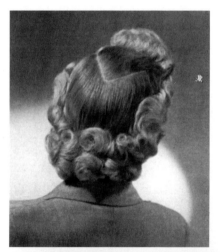

waves. The first wave should be combed in and its ends curled away from the face. The second wave should then be combed in and ends should be curled in two rows of alternating directions.
3. The back hair is pin curled up and away from the center back of the head.

COMB OUT
Brush the hair smooth and push the waves into place. Slightly fluff out the back hair.

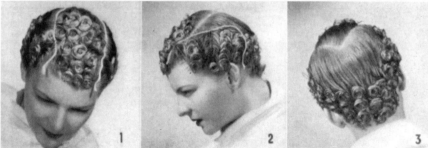

HIGH COMMAND, Circa 1943

Hairstyle By Thomas Frank

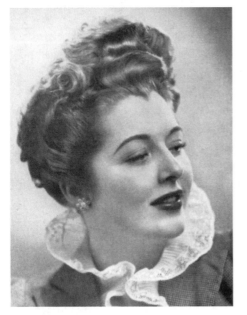

High waves end in soft casual curls and the entire hairstyle has an upward trend. The hair from the nape of the neck is swept up and forward. Large combs, hidden in the curls in back, keep the back hair in place.

SETTING INSTRUCTIONS

1. Create a side part on the right side of the head that extends from the forehead to the nape of the neck. Before any curls are made, the hair is combed sideways and up, away from the part, to help form the curls in back of the front and left sections. On the right side alternate directions of vertical rows of pin curls as in the photos below.
2. A full wave is set in the front with curled ends..
3. On the left side, the first vertical row of curls in set in a counterclockwise direction. The second row is set in a clockwise direction. The rest of the hair is set in rows of curls going in a counterclockwise direction.
4. When the set is dry, comb the top hair up and push the waves into place. Then comb the side up and back.

✺MODERN METHOD

Wave the sides and front with a waving iron and curl the ends and back with a curling iron.

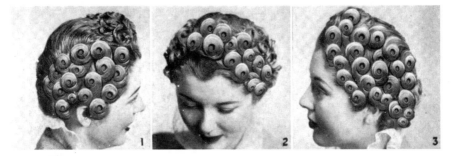

66

"Be the WOMEN behind the MAN behind the GUN"

THE WAR YEARS

Hairstyles during the war years changed drastically from what had been previously popular. The arrival of women into the service and work force required styles to change from being long and glamorous to being short, simple, and sophisticated.

With shorter styles in vogue, women went to great lengths to keep their styles looking feminine, which kept morale up, and the boys coming home. If a woman did not have naturally curly hair, permanent waves were the next best thing. Hair with a permanent wave could easily be styled for wartime work, and with a flick of a comb, quickly modified for evening glamour.

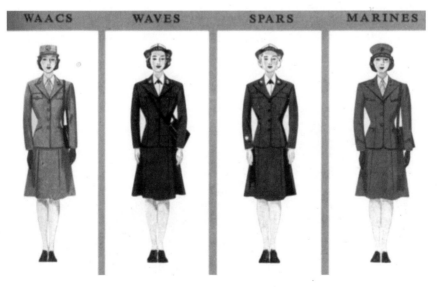

| WAACS | WAVES | SPARS | MARINES |

Having the haircut three inches in length seemed to be most popular during the war years. This length, when styled correctly, provided ample room above the collar (for service gals) while still long enough to maintain a feminine appearance. However, haircuts ranged from severe shortness at about 2 inches in length (that a woman might receive at service headquarters) to a more styleable four-inch length.

Women that joined the service had to follow strict regulations regarding their hair. Hair had to be kept neat, and most importantly, above the

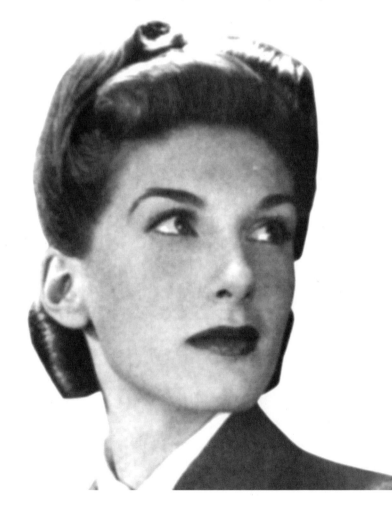

collar. Women could have their hair long or short. If kept long (which was very rare), the hair was pinned up or curled under in such a way that kept it above the collar. Women working in factory jobs, had to be concerned with safety. Most cut their hair or tied it back with bandannas and scarves.

Service regulations led the way to what would be called the "Victory Haircut." The "Victory Haircut" was a general term to describe short, 2 – 3 inch long haircuts, which were adopted by the majority of the women. Even career gals with their extremely tailored suits donned the short look that not only fit with the tailored suit, but assured their support for the war effort.

Although some women did keep their hair long, this chapter concentrates on the shorter styles of the war years. Medium length and longer styles during these years can found elsewhere throughout the book.

Military Tactics

At best, the war against the Axis powers is a grim affair, and will command almost everyone's attention for some time to come. For the rigorous life ahead during which every day will be packed with action and little attention can be allotted to fussy hairdos, Robert Fiance of New York has given us four short, simple and practical hairstyle designs. Each will require well-shaped hair, cut from three to five inches. Soft permanents assure their success.

FLIGHT COMMAND

Up on the sides, in a beautiful pompadour movement. It's sleek and fitted across the back to bring out a lovely natural "V" shape at the neckline. Four rows of sculptured curls are turned in alternate directions on top. The sides are shaped off the face and two rows of curls are turned forward. The back is swept across and up, then set in large flat curls. See Right.

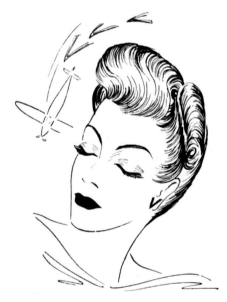

MANEUVER

Retreats off the face on the sides, down in back, with pert bangs on the forehead. The sides consist of three rows of sculptured curls turned back and up from the face. The back is combed down and to one side and is finished off in soft curls. Hair should be about five inches in length all over the head. See Right.

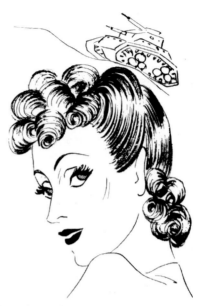

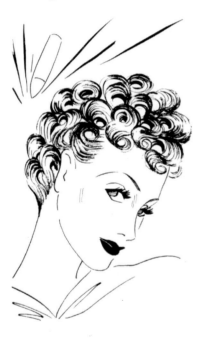

BOMBSHELL

An arrangement of short, short hair that "splatters" and curls up all over the head. Large, well formed, sculptured curls are set all over the head. On the sides the curls should be turned off the face. All of the hair is about 3 ½ to 4 inches long. See Left.

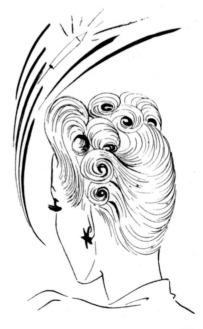

ROCKET

Up-up off the face, sweeping around the back and finishing off in a soft array of curls on top of the head. The top is set in pompadour curls. The sides are shaped off the face and set in rows of sculptured curls. Back is snug and firm across the head, finished off with a well-placed comb hidden by the curls on the side. See right.

FOUR STAR HAIRDO, CIRCA 1943

Hairstyle by Albert of Fifth Avenue

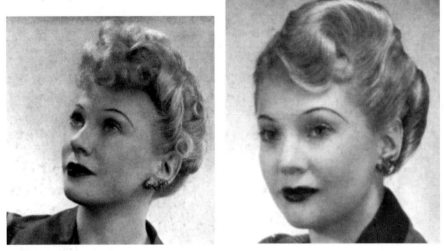

This style can be re-combed into two different versions – smooth or soft – depending on the wearers mood and the occasion. Styled for 3 – 4 inch hair.

Set hair as in illustrations. When dry comb out the hair and style. Comb smoothly for a sleek military style or fluff the bangs forward for a more casual factory worker style.

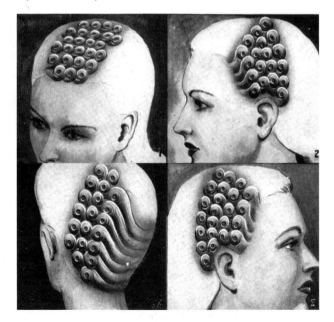

FEATHEREDGE INFORMALITY, CIRCA 1943

This hairstyle's ease and manageability was mainly worn by defense plant workers. The hair is two to three inches in length and parted on the side down the back of the head. The crown is combed smooth and all hair is set in pin curls curling towards the back of the head. When the curls dry, brush them out just a bit, making sure to keep the middle of the back of the head smooth and neat. Very "Shirley Temple-esque"

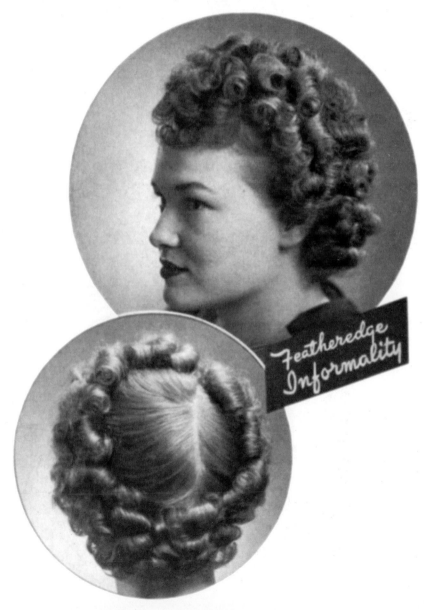

DOUBLE DUTY STRATEGY, CIRCA 1942

Hairstyle by Berthold

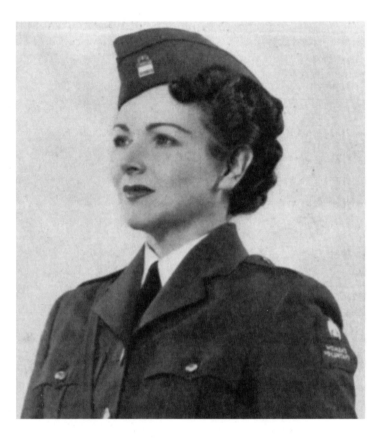

"Miss Daly's hair is three inches long – the approved length for women in uniform since the hair should not touch the collar – and the style has the dual advantage of being crisp and business like while it retains a definite air of flattering femininity."

PIN CURLS SETTING GUIDE

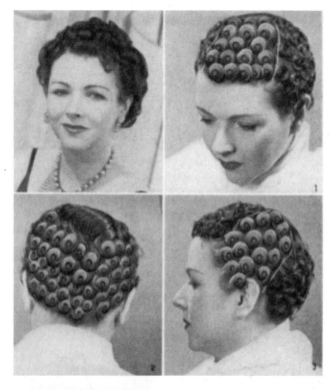

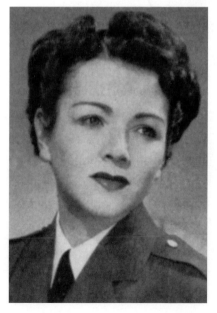

SETTING INSTRUCTIONS

1. The curls on the top are all wound counterclockwise.
2. On the side the pin curls alternate between clockwise and counterclockwise.
3. The back is combed down in a diagonal shadow wave and the ends are pin curled.

Note: This style may be modified and recombed to suit the individual.

POMPOM CURLCUT, CIRCA 1942

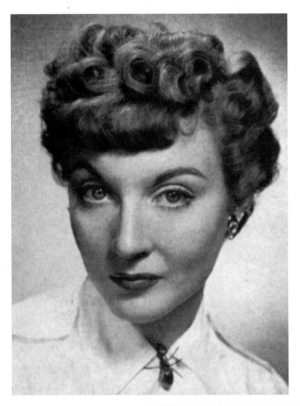

"For defense work, it may be worn with the new Defense shirt showing shoulder epaulets – creating the tailored effect. Hair should be cut fairly short and top hair should fall just above the eyebrows."

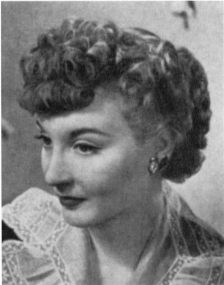

Defend that Permanent

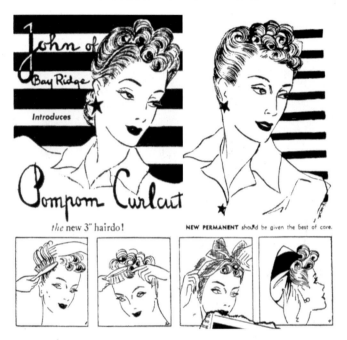

SETTING INSTRUCTIONS

1.   Set all hair in pin curls going in a backward direction from the face.

2.   Set the top hair the same way except for the first row near the hairline. Set that row in pin curls coming forward over the forehead.

3.   The back hair is set in tons of pin curls.

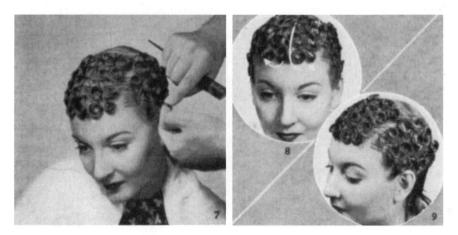

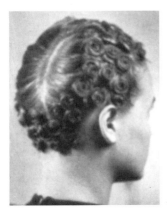

DEFENSE PLANT,
CIRCA 1942

A perfectly feminine hairstyle that is very easy to style and upkeep. The hair should be three inches in length.

SETTING INSTRUCTIONS:
1. Part the hair in back in an elongated cowlick part.
2. Curl the rest of the hair away from the part.

COMB OUT
Brush the curls out. Reform and define curls around your finger. They should stay in place without much worry. The curls may be secured in place with hair pins if extra support is needed.

VARIATION
Using the same setting for hair that is four to five inches in length and parted straight down the back. Top hair should be combed out into puff curls.

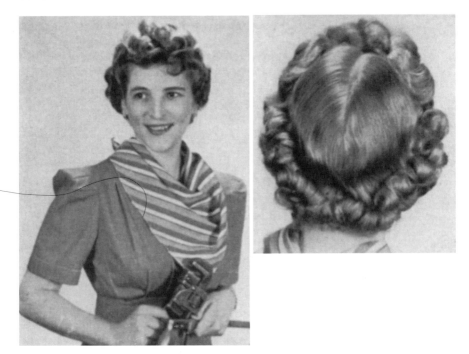

CHAPTER FIVE

FORMAL AND UP-DOs

PERIOD UP-DOs

The most important part of a 1940s period up-do is that the back and sides are pinned up. 1940s up-dos concentrate on having height towards the front of the head instead of at the back. The back can be pinned up using any method as long as it looks clean, uncluttered, and does not detract from the rest of the hairstyle.

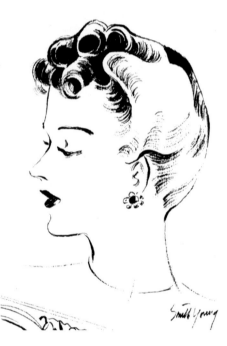

HEADLINE FOR SPRING, Circa 1943
Hairstyle by Frank Ort

"A 'quick change' coif, that can be combed in either 'up' or 'down' lines, depending on the mood of the wearer or the occasion. Very popular for the new spring hats. The up-do version has waved sides brushed up, secured back hair pinned up, and a cluster of curls on the top portion of the head."

Hair may be set by following the numbered illustrations.

MODERN METHOD
Lightly wave the sides with a waving iron and pin up. Brush up the back, as in the illustrations, and secure with pins. Barrel curl all of the top hair and pin in place without combing out the curls.

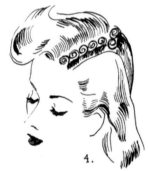

1.

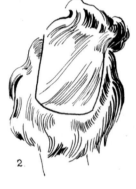

2.

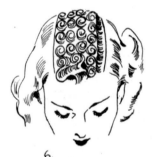

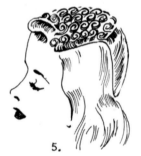

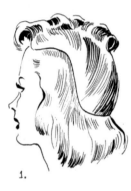

4.

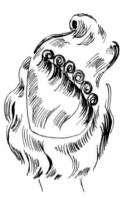

5.

6.

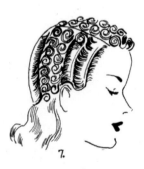

7.

8.

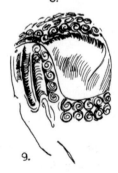

9.

SUCCESSFUL VERSION UP-DO, Circa 1942

Hairstyle by Sidney Guilaroff

This style was designed for the piquant, girlish beauty of young Laraine Day. The back hair is swept upward, ending in a large puff roll atop the head. The front is combed forward in a crisply waved bang fastened with a dainty ribbon. Another version at the right, shows the style trimmed with ostrich tips and the front combed into little ringlets.

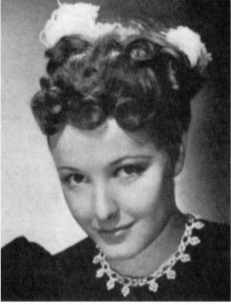

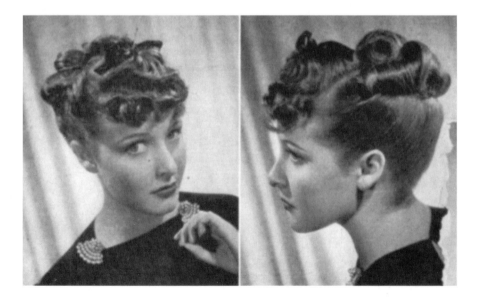

FORMAL UP HAIRSTYLE WITH FLUFF BANGS

Set the top hair into pin curls for fluff bangs. Gather up side hair into high reverse rolls. The back and crown hair is gathered into a flat roll right behind where the flower will be. When the hair dries, fluff out the bangs and place a flower between the bangs and the flat roll in back.

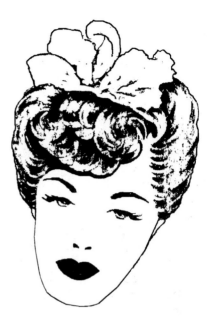

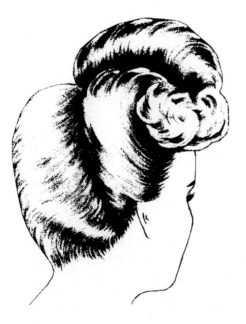

BACK DIAGONAL PART

The top hair is set in a half wave reverse roll. Pin curl bangs above the right eye and fluff out when dry. The back is parted diagonally. The top half of the back hair combines with the side hair and is folded into a flat roll. The bottom half of the back hair is combined with the left side hair and also folded into a flat roll.

SYMPHONY, Circa 1943

The perfect up-do created for easy to handle short hair. The ideal compliment to the smart simplicity of early 1940s evening gowns and dinner dresses. Hair should be four to six inches long all over the head in order to replicate this style.

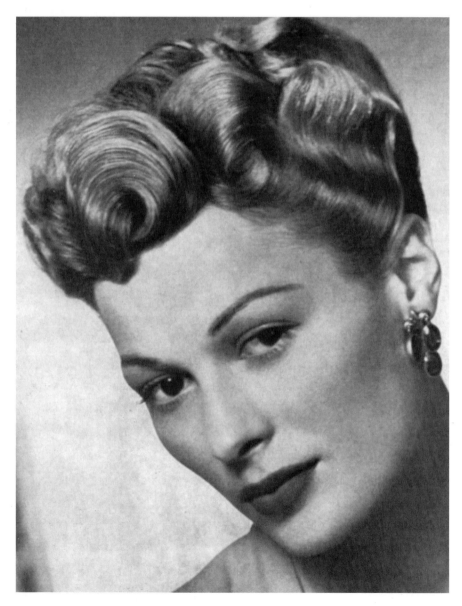

SETTING INSTRUCTIONS

1. Part top hair as indicated in illustration and wind curls in a counterclockwise direction. Leave the curls open in the center.
2. Create a full wave on each side of the head and pin curl the ends.
3. Imagine a straight line going down the back of the head and mold the pin curls up and away from it, see illustration.

COMB OUT

Brush the sides smooth and up towards the crown. Push waves into hair. Each side of the back hair should be brushed up and toward the imaginary center-line. Top hair should be brushed out and formed into puffs and pinned securely.

FOR LONG HAIR

Arrange the front as shown. The sides and back would be set as shown and then pinned up.

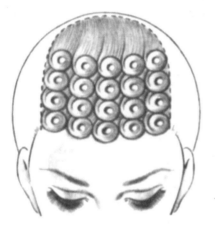

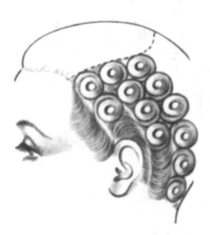

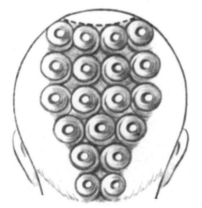

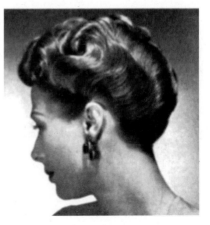

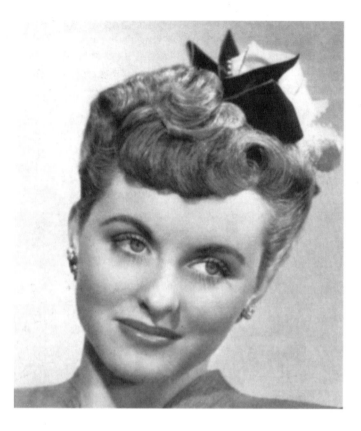

CHERYL WALKER, Circa 1943

Star of "Stage Door Canteen"

The sides are waved and swept back and up from the hairline. The back
is combed up into a modified up-do. Soft curls are allowed to fall into
bangs on the forehead and the whole hairdo is topped off with a hair
bow attached above the bangs. This style is easy to comb and stays neatly
in place with almost no effort. To keep the up-swept hair in place, hairpins
are tucked into the curls in back.

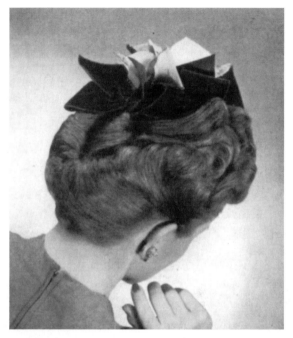

SETTING INSTRUCTIONS

1. In the top section, the first and third rows are wound clockwise, and the second and fourth rows are wound counterclockwise.

2. On the left side, the hair is set in five vertical rows of curls. The first and fourth rows are wound clockwise, and the second, third, and fifth are wound counterclockwise.

3. On the right side the hair is set in four rows of vertical curls. The first row is set counterclockwise and the rest of the rows are set clockwise.

4. The back is set in five vertical rows of curls. The two rows on the right are wound clockwise, and the three rows on the left are wound counterclockwise.

5. When dry, comb out and style.

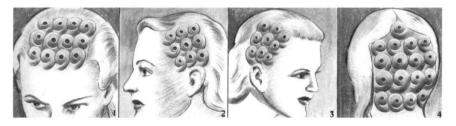

TWO ROLLS

A very easy way to create a formal hairstyle is to part the hair on the side and make two reverse rolls coming in towards the part. How much hair you use in each roll and the amount of backcombing you do, will affect the height and volume of the finished hairstyle. There are two examples shown on this page, that use the same set, but are styled differently.

For both styles, start with the hair parted on the side. On the smaller side create a reverse roll. On the larger side, combine the top hair and side hair to make one large reverse roll.

For the example below left, the back hair is left down and the ends are curled.

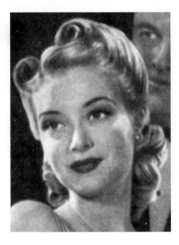

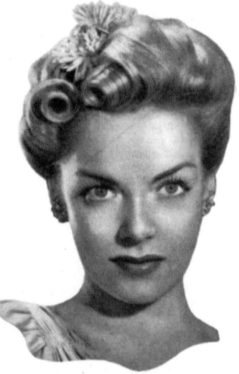

In the example to the right, much more hair has been used for each roll and much more backcombing has been applied. The back hair is pinned up and a flower is secured in between the two rolls.

PILES OF CURLS

This is a very easy up-do to do. All the hair is set in pin curls or curlers. Once curls have been set and dried, softly brush out the hair to slightly separate the curls. Pin up the back and sides by securing hair with a circle of bobbie pins around the head. Make sure to cover bobbie pins with over hanging curls pinned in place. Pile curls on top of head and secure with bobbie pins if needed. For more defined curls on top of the head, roll pieces over a round handle of a brush, or around your finger, and pin in place. Allow a few small curls to dangle on the forehead.

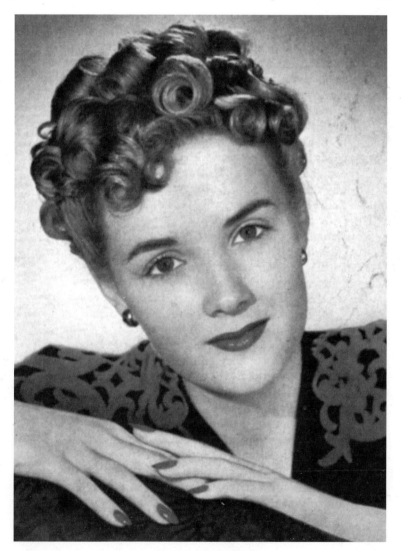

CHAPTER SIX

HAIR ACCESSORIES

BRAIDS

Although popular throughout the decade, braids and braided pieces really came into vogue during the mid 1940s. They were crossed in front over the head, brought up at each side of the head from a center back part, crossed over the nape of the neck to soften the hairline, used high to make a coronet, and as always...parted down the center and left to hang with ribbons attached to the ends.

PIGTAILS, CIRCA 1941
"Once upon a time girls outgrew their pigtails; now they think it's fun to go back to them. Add a velvet bow to the ends for interest. For blondes try black velvet; for brunettes, bright shades."

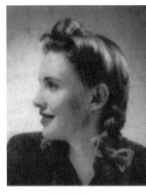

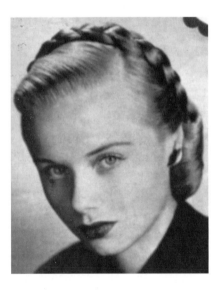

BRAIDED PIECE, CIRCA 1947
A braided piece added to a shoulder length bob creates a different look in no time. The hair is parted on the side and brushed smooth. The braid is set across the head and secured with bobbie pins.

DIFFERENT COLORS, CIRCA 1943
A very fun look from 1943 is to add a braided hairpiece the exact opposite of your natural coloring. Blondes and red heads would use brown and black, respectively. Brunettes would use a blond braid.

CROSSED BRAIDS

This is a great braid variation. Make reverse rolls for the front and side hair. Take the back hair starting directly behind the ears and make two braids. Criss-cross and loop each braid, pin at the nape of the neck. Tie a ribbon around where the braids intersect for a cute touch.

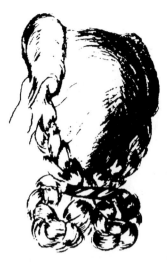

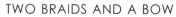

TWO BRAIDS AND A BOW

Make a reverse roll for the front hair. Comb the back hair forward and up toward the temples. Make a braid on both sides. Tie braids at nape of neck with ribbon or bow.

QUEENLY CORONET, CIRCA 1944

For evening importance, a variation on the queenly coronet. A false braid is used, divided two ways instead of three and twisted over and over with strings of pearls to make a coil. For the basic hairdo, part the hair straight through the center, comb it up and off the face and brush into reverse rolls. A ribbon may be substituted for pearls if you prefer.

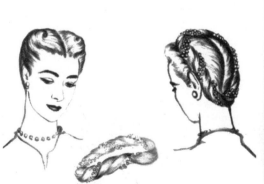

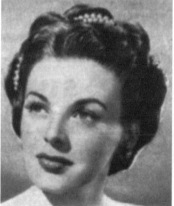

RIBBONS AND BOWS

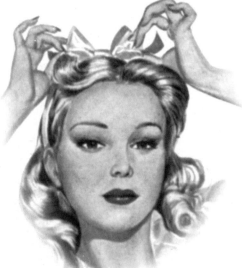

The use of ribbons and bows really can turn any hairdo into a more fun or formal do. A correctly placed bow makes any hairstyle sweet and becoming.

If you're in a hurry a small ribbon can be tied around the head with a bow on top to create a really cute hairdo.

RIBBON OR BANDS WITH PEOPLES NAMES

One fad started by college girls in the early 1940s was to wear ribbons with their boyfriend's name on them tied in their hair. To replicate this fad, you can buy ribbon with the name already printed on, stitch the name into the ribbon yourself, paint it on using acrylics, or write it on using a special fabric marker.

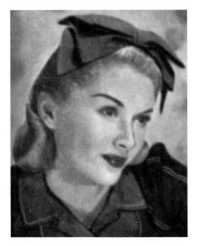

LARGE BOW, CIRCA 1944

A large bow is worn on the top of the head in hat fashion. The rest of the hair is kept smooth and pulled back from the face.

SNOODS & HAIRNETS

Snoods were used to keep the back hair neat for women with medium to long length hair. The front and side hair was usually done up in rolls or waves, while the back hair was curled or rolled under and kept in place by the snood. Snoods came in different thicknesses. Thick, loose-knit snoods were considered much more casual than thin, lightweight snoods (looks almost like a thick hairnet).

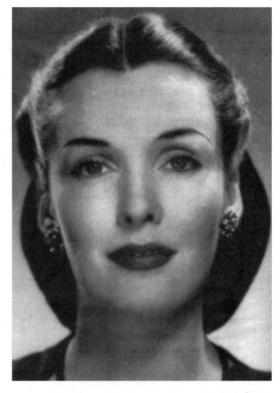

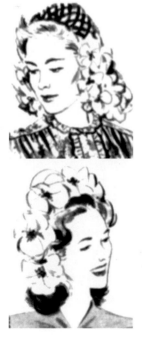

A different option was using netting to keep the hair in place. For more formal or fancy hairstyles, instead of using snoods, women of the 1940s would use invisible hairnets. Hairnets were used to keep the back hair neat and were almost invisible when used. Because they were barely noticeable, they were considered more sleek and sophisticated.

For fun party looks, both snoods and hairnets were decorated with flowers, ribbons, and bows.

Snoods and hairnets can still be purchased today if you'd like to replicate this look. Besides being accessories, both snoods and hairnets may be used to keep your set tight and springy on your way to an event. Once you get to the event, take the net or snood off and you have fresh springy curls! Appendix B will tell you where to get 'em!

SCARVES AND TURBANS

Scarves and turbans can be used as decorative accessories and/or as utility pieces to keep the hair out of your face. Since scarves and turbans come in a variety of colors, patterns, sizes, and thicknesses they can easily be coordinated to match your outfit. This makes them both very versatile accessories.

SCARF HEADBAND
A scarf tied up and around the nape of the neck will keep the hair back and neat for sporting events. See Right.

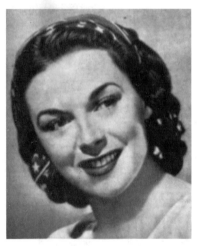

SCARF TRICK, CIRCA 1944
The scarf trick is an easy practical way to control hair neatly for active sports and keeps the hair off the neck during hot summer days. Make a full-length center part and divide the hair into two strands at each side behind the ears. Fold a large square scarf diagonally and arrange headband fashion across the front of the head. Braid scarf ends with strands of hair. Bring braids together at nape of neck and tie scarf ends in a pert bow.

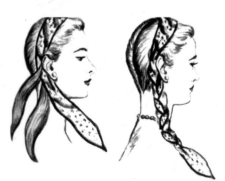

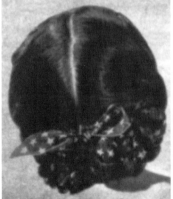

MAKE YOUR OWN TURBAN!

You'll need a fabric of soft wool, a wool jersey, or a very firmly woven rayon crepe. A yard of 40-inch material will make two turbans. Cut the turban 36-inches long and half the width of material. Fold at A and seam the folded end. With a series of gathers, gather this seam into a 2½-inch measure. Place the gathered material at the beginning of your hairline in the center front, mark the turban, as shown in B. Split the unfinished end through the center of the fabric up to the mark on the material, so that the ends can cross and wrap around the head. Tie the turban and make sure you have split it so it ties at the most becoming angle. When the effect is just what you want, hem the unfinished edges.

ROSIE STYLE

A scarf tying the hair back a la Rosie the Riveter.

Taking a square scarf, fold in half to make a triangle shape. Place the long, straight folded edge across the nape of the neck. Bring the two longer corners up towards the forehead and the shorter center corner up over the crown. Tie the two longer corner together trying to knot in the center corner. Pin in place to secure if needed. This is also a great cover up while your hair is in a pin curl set.

FLOWERS & OTHER INTERESTING THINGS

Flowers can be used to liven up any hairdo, add color, and camouflage hairstyling mistakes. The use of real or silk flowers depends on what look you're going for. Real flowers are by far the most beautiful but tend to wilt rather quickly. If you can find a variety that holds up well, you should use them. Otherwise silk is the next best thing.

Silk flowers can either look really fake or really good. Try to find flowers that look as real as possible and are medium in size.

NOTE
The most important thing regarding flower placement is to try and create balance in the hairstyle. It just looks bad if flowers are sticking out sideways from your head. On the following pages are a few ideas for flower use and placeage.

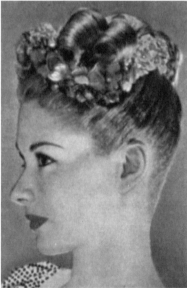

EVENING HAIRDO FOR SPRING, CIRCA 1945
Hair is swept up into barrel rolls on top. Then an adorable hairdo gadget is wound around the rolls. The gadget is wired ribbon, bent into shape, then covered with flowers. Wire ribbon can be found at fabric and craft stores. Silk flowers can be sewn on or hot glued.

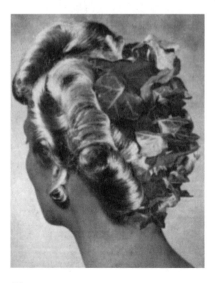

FALL LEAVES
Silk leaves can be attached with bobbie pins to the back of a hairstyle to add back interest. Great idea for a fall season look. You can modify this look for the Christmas season by replacing the leaves with poinsettias. See Left.

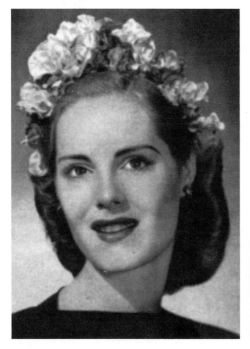

HEADBAND
Transform a daytime do into a nighttime do in seconds! Attach your favorite silk flowers to a headband with a hot glue gun. You can make sure to attach enough flowers so you cover the band completely, or attach flowers only at the sides of the headband close to the ears. Wherever you decide to place the flowers, make sure they look balanced and neat. See Left.

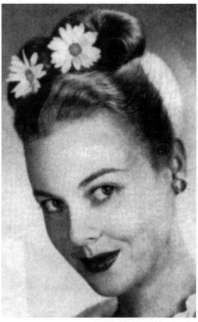

ROMANTIC SUMMER DO, CIRCA 1945
Gently waved at the temples and topped with curls. This works best for hair about six inches long with a natural curl or good permanent. Secure real or silk daisies in the hair to complete the look. See Right.

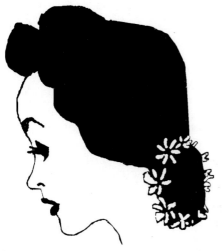

FLOWERS TUCKED INTO ROLLS OR KNOTS
Try tucking flowers into rolls or knots at the nape of the neck. Make a roll at the nape of the neck or a knot of short curls tied together in back. Pin small flowers around the roll or knot. See Left.

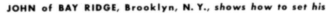

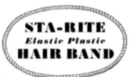

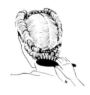
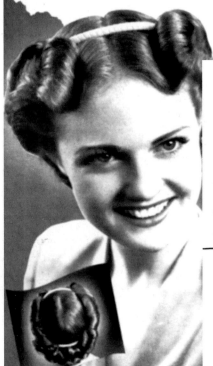
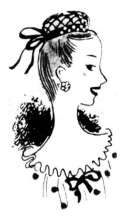

FAT LITTLE BRIOCHE, CIRCA 1945
"It's mew to slick your hair up into a fat little brioche (that's French for bun!) and snare it in a tiny net. An elastic band holds the updo up. A glittery choker borrowed from your necklace drawer conceals mechanism, adds a bit of chi-chi."

PROBLEM SOLVER
Q + A

Question: Do I need to get a vintage haircut to create a period style?
Answer: Although a period haircut will make it easier to create vintage styles, you do not need to have one. The most important thing is to have layers in your hair that you can work with.

Question: If I get a period haircut, do I have to always style my hair period?
Answer: No. A period haircut is really just a shaped layered cut. Having layers allows you to easily style your hair modern or period.

Question: What do I need to hold my hair in place and keep it up?
Answer: Hair combs and crinkled bobbie pins seem to work the best.

Question: I would like to know in what direction to set pin curls for a pompadour with a wave in it. My pompadours never come out with a wave in them.
Answer: Pin curl the first row of hair in the direction the hair falls naturally ½ inch over the hairline on the forehead. See to it that all the curls are even, perfectly round, and flat. Wind all of the other rows in the opposite direction. For wider waves alternate direction every two rows. When combing out the pompadour, brush out the curls first. Then from the back of the pompadour, comb the hair forward up and over the forehead. Backcomb the back of the pompadour to add height. Then comb the front back and up in one sweeping motion. The wave should fall easily into place.

Question: What is the MacArthur hairdress?
Answer: (From American Hairdresser, Circa 1942):
A MacArthur hairdress is kept quite short and simple all over the head, similar to the general's own hair cut.

Question: The curls at my neckline never come out very curly. How do I fix it?
Answer: Curls at the neckline fail most often because they are loosely set. To make these curls tighter and more lasting, wind the end hairs on a stick. You can use the end of a pencil or pen as a stick to wind the hair around. Wind the hair around the stick, as shown in the photo. To make the curl "stick" and to eliminate fishhooks, reverse the direction of the stick after the curl has been made. This method is great for getting tight curls into straight hair.

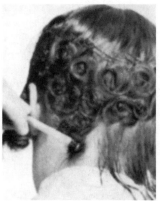

Question: Before I set or style my hair should it be clean or dirty?
Answer: This really depends on what type of hair you have. If you are doing a quick style with hot rollers, curling irons, etc, it is sometimes better to have slightly dirty hair. We're not talking crusty, but more like day-old hair. If you have ample time to set your hair in real curlers or pin curls, it's always best to start out with setting lotion added to clean, damp hair.

Question: Do I have to cut my hair short if I'm trying to achieve a military look?
Answer: No. Just find a way to pin the hair up or secure it so it is above the collar.

Question: What is a Victory Hair Cut?
Answer: From American Hairdresser, Circa 1943
"For the Victory Hair Cut, the hair is cut about two to three inches in length depending, of course, upon the type of person. A permanent wave is given in the usual fashion. Pin or sculpture curl in a cartwheel fashion. When dry, comb to suit the face and neck." See Below.

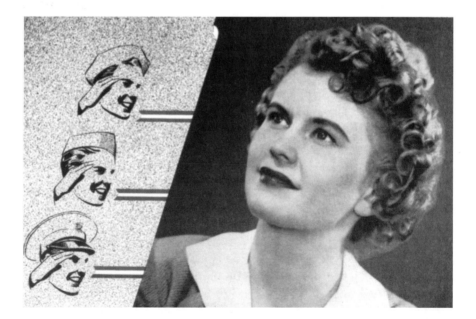

BACK INTEREST

Many women concentrate just on the front of the hair and forget the back needs special attention also. The illustrations on this page show what the back hair should look like versus what's usually done (shown in photographs).

Many things can cause the back hair to look frizzy and dull these include:

• Curls that are too tight.
Solution: Make larger curls.

• Hair that does not hold curl well.
Solution: Use a setting lotion or get a perm.

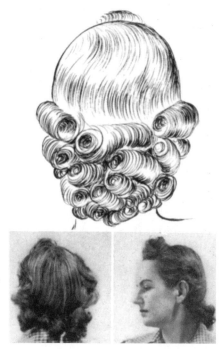

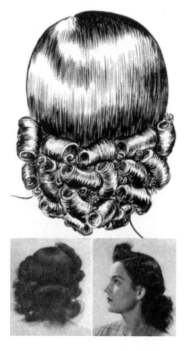

• Curl is brushed right out of hair.
Solution: Don't brush the hair so much.

• Formation of the curls is not tight enough or badly done.
Solution: Practice your curling methods.

• Hair is too heavy and needs a haircut.
Solution: Get a good, layered haircut.

• The hair needs layers and or is cut badly.
Solution: Get a better cut or shorter layers.

• The hair is damaged, dry and unhealthy.
Solution: Use a conditioner and setting lotion.

APPENDIX A
1940S BEAUTY SUPPLY
TOOL KIT

Your 1940s beauty supply tool kit should include the following items:

BOBBIE PINS
To pin hair elements in place like rolls and pompadours. Straight Bobbie Pins - Great for women with thick hair. I have thin hair and these never work for me. They always seem to slide out on their own. Kinked Bobbie Pins - Great for all hair types. These hold better than the straight bobbie pins in thinner hair.

BOWS, RIBBONS, AND SCARVES
Make sure to have plenty of bows, ribbons, and scarves on hand. If you're running out the door and don't have time for a full hairstyle, tie a cute "Minnie Mouse" bow in your hair in seconds flat. Scarves can be used "Rosie the Riveter" - style to get hair out of the way quickly or to keep pin curls in place while drying.

BRUSH

Get a good brush for brushing out curls into smooth waves and making curls fluff out without fizzing.

COMB

A comb is used to create clean parts and to tease the hair for rolls and pompadours.

CURLERS / ROLLERS

Curlers or hot rollers can be used to curl hair instead of using pin curls

CURLING IRON

Creates curl in the hair by using heat. Great for quick fixes.

HAIRNET

Get an invisible hairnet the same color as your hair. It can be used to keep up the small nape hair tidy in an up hairstyle. It can also be pinned around a hair roll at the nape of the neck to keep the hair neat and tidy.

HAIRSPRAY

Hairspray is necessary as a finishing spray. Never use it to keep rolls and pompadours in place. Rolls and pompadours should be pinned in place securely and then hairsprayed to control any loose hairs. If you'll be doing lots of dancing or vigorous activity, hairspray the base of the roll, pompadour, or wave for extra security making sure not to create too much stiffness.

MARCEL WAVE CLIPS

Although it is generally recommended to use a comb when setting waves, Marcel wave clips come in handy for women, like myself, with

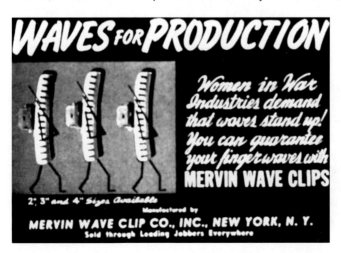

stick straight hair that have no natural bend to their hair. These clips create a very strong edge that doesn't even compare to comb-waved hair, but can be used as a last resort.

These clips are also great for refreshing waves

in dry hair if you've brushed the hair out too much and lost the wave ridges.

MARCEL WAVE IRON
Used to create waves in the hair using heat. Works like a crimping iron, but makes deeper waves. Big bucks!

PIN CURL CLIPS
Pin curl clips are flat clips that hold the pin curl in place without leaving indentations in the curl. I use these extensively. They are mush easier to manage and are much less time consuming than bobbie pins.

POMADE
Pomade is generally used as a controlling agent and can add shine to the hair without adding stiffness. It's great for women with thick hair. But on thin hair it tends to look greasy.

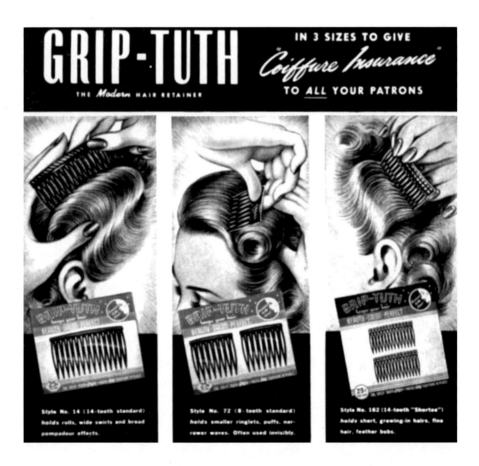

RAT

A foam tube usually inserted into a roll to create extra volume. You will need a rat if you have very fine or thin hair that does not create ample volume when teased.

SETTING LOTION

Setting lotion is the key factor to keeping curl in your hair. I've tried many of them. Since I have straight hair, I've found that the ones that work best on me are the ones that are manufactured for women of color.

SNOOD

Snoods are knitted bags that keep curls and hair in place. They are generally used for medium long to long length hair.

APPENDIX B
WHERE TO FIND BEAUTY SUPPLIES

Most of the beauty supplies are pretty easy to come by in any city. For those of you that live out in the boonies, your local beauty supply store should be able to order hard-to-get beauty items for you.

BEAUTY SUPPLY STORES
Most any town or city has at least one beauty supply store. If your town is not fortunate enough to have a beauty store catering to women of color you might have to search online for mail order companies and manufacturers. Every beauty shop will carry combs, brushes, curling irons, waving irons, both straight and narrow bobbie pins, pomades, shine enhancers, etc. You should also be able to find a good quality hairspray that will not flake off. Ask the sales associate to recommend a hairspray for your hair type that will hold strongly, but not stiffen the hair.

Beauty stores that cater to women of color usually have all the staples, plus more. If you don't want to make two trips, you can pick up all of your staple items while shopping for your setting lotion. I usually purchase my setting lotion, pin curl clips, marcel wave clips, hairnets, and snoods all at the same time. They usually have a selection of fun turbans and scarves to wear while your hair is up in pin curls. Ask the sales associates what setting lotion would be best for your hair type and texture. I tend to like the setting lotions that foam up. I bought a large bottle that will last me forever and paid around $3.00.

CRAFT STORES

I love craft stores. At craft stores you can find silk and dried flowers to beautify any 1940s hairstyle. Craft stores almost always carry ribbon. So if you can't find the right color, size, and fabric type at your local fabric shop, try a craft store before loosing hope. Another great thing about craft stores is they carry seasonal decorations. For Autumn, I found great velvet maple leaves to pin into my rolls. During the winter months try searching for holly or mistletoe to put in your hair. In spring bright flowers and for summer months, simplicity and casualness are most important. A sun flower tucked into a simple roll at the nape of the neck looks clean and fresh.

FABRIC STORES

Most fabric stores are apt to carry a large selection of ribbons and bows. Go through your wardrobe and figure out the basic ribbon colors that you need to go with your everyday outfits. Plan on getting ribbon that is a little more special for dates and special occasions. Most of the time you can get a whole roll of ribbon for around $4.00. Use the excess ribbon to accent snoods or braids. If you'd rather do without the excess ribbon, you can usually buy pieces. Always make sure to buy a yard so you can have a little excess at the ends.

VINTAGE CLOTHING STORES, THRIFT STORES

You should scout out your local vintage clothing store for fine vintage scarves. Look for vintage prints that are fun and in good condition. If your vintage clothing store does not have a wide selection, your local thrift store should have tons of pretty scarves to choose from.

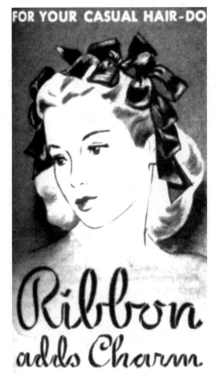

FOR YOUR CASUAL HAIR-DO

Ribbon adds Charm.

INDEX
WHERE TO FIND HAIRSTYLES FOR YOUR HAIR LENGTH

LONG LENGTH HAIR
Shoulder length or longer.

CASUAL
48, 49, 52-57

WORKING GIRL
62, 63

FORMAL & UP-DO'S
80-85, 88, 89

MEDIUM LENGTH HAIR
Chin length to shoulder length.
CASUAL
46-51

WORKING GIRL
62-65, 71

FORMAL & UP-DO'S
80-85, 88, 89

SHORT HAIR
Chin length or shorter.
CASUAL
43-45

WORKING GIRL
61, 64, 66, 70-71, 72-78

FORMAL & UP-DO'S
84, 86, 89

GET THE SCOOP!

Wanna find out about upcoming vintage living projects before anyone else?

Copy or tear off the bottom portion of this page and send it in to be included on our mailing list for FREE.

You'll get information and discounts on upcoming titles and don't worry ... we won't sell or give your info away.

Yes, please put me on your mailing list!

Name _____

Address_____

Email _____

Cut out along dotted line and send to:
Streamline Press - Research Division
2106 Albury Avenue
Long Beach, CA 90815

Letting us know what you're interested in will help us get it to you!

I'm interested in books about (check all that apply):

☐ ALL OF THE BELOW

☐ Victorian Beauty and Hairstyles ☐ Victorian Fashion
☐ Edwardian Beauty and Hairstyles ☐ Edwardian Fashion
☐ 1920s Beauty and Hairstyles ☐ 1920s Fashion
☐ 1930s Beauty and Hairstyles ☐ 1930s Fashion
☐ 1940s Beauty and Hairstyles ☐ 1940s Fashion
☐ 1950s Beauty and Hairstyles ☐ 1950s Fashion
☐ Other Eras Beauty and Hairstyles ☐ Other Eras Fashion
   please specify_____ please specify_____

☐ Other not listed here. Please specify_____
_____